WILL
IT
HURT?

A Parent's Practical Guide
to Children's Surgery

Will It Hurt?
A Parent's Practical Guide to Children's Surgery
Copyright © 2008 by Armen G. Ketchedjian, MD
Published by Warren Enterprises, LLC

For further information, please visit:
www.drketch.com

Printed in Unites States of America

Will It Hurt?
A Parent's Practical Guide to Children's Surgery
Armen G. Ketchedjian, M.D.
1. Title 2. Author 3. Medical

Library of Congress Control Number: 2008921845

ISBN-10: 0-9815373-0-8
ISBN-13: 978-0-9815373-0-6

617.98

WILL
IT
HURT?

A Parent's Practical Guide
to Children's Surgery

By Armen G. Ketchedjian, MD
("Dr. Ketch")

Warren Enterprises, LLC

This guide would not be possible without the inspiration from Denise Ketchedjian. She gave me the idea while I was working on the adult version of the guide. She urged me to start working on *Will It Hurt?* immediately, to help spare thousands of parents the anxiety associated with their children's surgery and help children go through their procedures more easily.

I am extremely grateful for my close friend, Dr. Maxamillian Hartmannsgruber, whom I highly admire. He is an associate professor of anesthesia at NYU Medical School. I am thankful, on behalf of all the parents who will read my book, to Dr. Hartmannsgruber for providing his valuable time and tireless devotion to helping children and parents cope with the process of surgery.

I am also thankful to Mr. Robert Lucas for his contribution. He is quite talented as a physician's assistant in the field of aesthetics, deftly wielding a scalpel or a needle. I am more thankful for his talents as a wordsmith—he suggested the title of this guide.

A Note From Dr. Ketch

It is important to read this information prior to reading any portion in *Will It Hurt? A Parent's Practical Guide to Children's Surgery*. The information in this guide is intended as a supplement to, not a substitute for, the expertise and judgment of a healthcare professional. The information is not intended to cover all possible uses, directions, precautions, or permutations, circumstances, medical conditions, surgical procedures of what may or may not occur in actual clinical care or treatment.

- The information is provided as-is, and Dr. Armen Ketchedjian ("Dr. Ketch"), the publisher or anyone else associated with this guide does not warrant that it is complete, accurate or up to date.

- Non-healthcare professionals should consult their physicians before altering their treatment regimens and must follow medical treatment as directed by healthcare professionals who have assumed full responsibility of care.

- Dr. Armen G. Ketchedjian ("Dr. Ketch"), the publisher or anyone else associated with this guide are not in any way liable for misuse, misunderstanding or injuries resulting from any treatment or outcome.

This is only a guide and is not a replacement for treatment. Your healthcare provider's advice and treatment will always supersede any advice or guidance contained within this guide. If you have any questions, you must consult with your healthcare provider immediately.

—Dr. Ketch

CONTENTS

Chapter 5: Finding the Right
Surgeon and the Right Place

Section II
PREPARING FOR SURGERY

Chapter 6: First Steps

Chapter 7: The Medical Team

Chapter 8: What the Surgeon
Has to Know Before Surgery

Chapter 9: Pre-surgery Procedures

Chapter 10: Understanding Anesthesia

Section III
THE ACTUAL OPERATION

Chapter 11: What to Expect

Chapter 12: Risks of Surgery in Children

Chapter 13: Allergies and Drug Sensitivity

Chapter 14: Blood Transfusions

Section IV
COMMONLY PERFORMED
PEDIATRIC SURGERIES

Chapter 15: General Guidelines

SPECIFIC PEDIATRIC SURGICAL PROCEDURES

Section V
BACK HOME

Chapter 16: Post-surgery Care
What You Should Be Concerned About After Surgery . 153

FOREWORD

I doubt there is a greater anxiety-building time or challenge for any parent than the illness of a child. That concern can become even greater if the child needs surgery.

I have seen the frustration and grief in the eyes of parents when confronted by their own limitations and fear in caring for their sick child. I have also seen the helplessness they feel as they hesitantly turn the care of their child over to the physicians and nurses—strangers, in a strange place, to both the parents and the child.

This feeling of helplessness can become even more difficult when the parents must leave the child pleading and crying, only to wait for what may seem like an eternity until they are able to see each other again in the recovery room. Parents can often feel pangs of guilt for allowing their child to go through this alone, without them. This is often the first time the child has been separated from his or her parents. It is entirely understandable why this may become a very anxious time for both parents and child.

The seriousness of a child's illness and the extensiveness of surgery definitely play direct roles in the level of parental anxiety. Every one of us handles stress differently and most parents, while distressed, remain calm. The occasional parent, who is obviously emotionally upset by the situation, will add to the anxiousness of an already stressful time, and everyone involved can become affected by this.

No words will ever remove the anxiety parents and children feel about an upcoming surgery or for that matter, the anxiety felt by anyone facing surgery. Therefore, I have written this book to help you and your child gain a clearer understanding of circumstances you will probably encounter in most hospitals for the majority of surgical procedures. By clarifying terms and addressing concerns often heard from parents before their child has surgery, I hope to make the experience a tiny bit smoother for you, the parent, and your child.

—*Armen G. Ketchedjian, MD*
   ("Dr. Ketch")

INTRODUCTION

"When we were children, we used to think that when we were grown-up we would no longer be vulnerable. But to grow up is to accept vulnerability. To be alive is to be vulnerable."
—Madeleine L'Engle,
Walking on Water: Reflections on Faith and Art

Children's healthcare needs are very different from those of adults and because of this, it is very important that their healthcare needs be provided by trained pediatric specialists who focus only on children. While most all parents agree with this, there are times during the life of a child when medical urgencies arise that can be overwhelming for families, and sometimes physicians, to manage. Most healthcare professionals agree that the safest and best possible outcome for each child is best ensured by a multi-disciplinary team approach that puts the child and parents at the center of care, surrounded by a team of experts who understand the very special needs in pediatric medicine and surgery.

According to Dr. Zeev Kain, the Chairman in the Department of Anesthesiology at the University of California at Irvine, "some 3 million children undergo anesthesia and surgery in the United States every year; 40 percent to 60 percent of these children develop significant behavioral stress prior to surgery."[1] Dr. Kain also stresses that "preoperative anxiety is associated with a number of poor postoperative outcomes."[2]

Navigating your way through the medical maze of hospitals and healthcare specialists who will manage a component of your child's care can be overwhelming for any parent. To provide you, the parent, with guidance in the management of that time in your life when your child will need surgery, and to help relieve some of your anxiety about the upcoming surgery, Dr. Ketchedjian has compiled this very extensive reference guide that will answer many of your questions and certainly provide enduring support to you and your family.

The pearls that Dr. Ketchedjian offers within this excellent guide are based on his own experiences in anesthesia over the past seventeen years; the experiences of his colleagues in anesthesia, surgery and other medical specialities; parents; and members of the healthcare team—all of who want to make your child's journey before, during and after surgery as seamless and as stress-free as possible.

---

[1]Kain ZN, Caldwell-Andrews A, Wang SH. Psychological preparation of the parent and pediatric surgical patient. Anesthesiol Clin North America. 2002;20:29-44.

[2]Kain ZN, Caldwell-Andrews AA. Preoperative psychological preparation of the child for surgery: an update. Anesthesiol Clin North America. 2005;23:597-614.

Section I

YOUR CHILD NEEDS SURGERY

Chapter 1
Getting the News

Your Initial Concerns

The News Is Overwhelming

This may be the first time since your child was born that you have heard these words from a physician: "Your child will need surgery." As the reality of this announcement begins to sink in, you may find yourself feeling more and more anxious about your child and more and more helpless in the situation that is beginning to unfold. You may be having trouble trying to understand when all of this began; you may be worrying about how you will get through it; and, you may be fighting the nagging feeling of fear, wondering, *Will my child be okay?*

What Do I Do first?

It will definitely help you to better cope with the situation if you can gain a deeper understanding of some of the medical reasons that surgery is now necessary for your child— you may feel better able to deal with the coming days ahead. Knowledge in any situation can ensure a better understanding of the process and the potential outcome—it will certainly help you feel more empowered in managing the surgery experience at the same time that you are comforting and reassuring your child.

Chapter 2
Now That You Know Your Child May Need Surgery

Compiling Your Child's Medical History

When visiting any physician always have pertinent medical information and necessary medical records with you. Despite the skill level and personable mannerisms of your child's surgeon, medical information can be lost or misplaced during transit from the pediatrician's office, or files kept off site can be misfiled. Your child's pediatrician cares for many children in his or her practice and he or she often reviews children's charts moments before seeing them in his or her office. In the event that the office staff appears to be having difficulty finding all of your child's records, you can help save precious time for the physician and yourself by providing the medical records yourself. Always carry your family medical history and your child's medical history with you when seeing a physician.

You may find it helpful to make your own notes ahead of time. Your child's surgeon may see two or three dozen patients in a day, and because of time constraints may appear rushed and have very little time to spend in conversation. By having all of your questions written in advance, you can help your physician to be efficient. Please also think about bringing toys and reading material to help distract your child if the wait for the pediatrician becomes longer than anticipated. Physicians are human beings prone to the same emotions that you are and while they are obligated to provide the same standard of care to all, there are situations that may require them to stay longer with a patient than initially thought.

Don't feel as though you need to purchase gifts for your physicians or shower them with compliments—do however, treat them professionally, respectfully and with kindness. You and your child's physician will experience a pleasant visit. It is rare in this day and age that basic etiquette is overlooked. Physicians are compassionate professionals in the business of

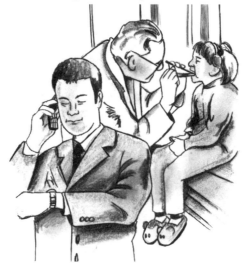

caring for people. Though this may sound incredibly simplistic to say, please show interest in the care of your child. Sometimes, a physician may be faced with an individual who has no interest in what is going on. While thankfully, this sort of behavior does not happen often, I've had patient interviews wherein the patient's parent was busy reading a book or magazine, or even chatting on a cell phone. As you can imagine, I was very surprised by the parent's level of disinterest.

This is the type of scenario that can create stress for the physician, the other members of the healthcare team and ultimately, the child. Try to remain very involved in the visit with the physician as he may mention something important you will want to remember at a later date. You may want to take notes at this time.

What Can I Expect to Happen Before the Surgery?

The Pre-operative Checkup

The pre-operative checkups that will be necessary will allow you and your surgeon opportunities to discuss the benefits and risks of the surgical procedure on behalf of your child. Depending on the complexity of the procedure, there will be many factors that come into play, including:

- Blood transfusions, which may play a role if the surgery is prolonged and complex, and involves organs and large blood vessels. Cell saver technology is often utilized to help conserve blood and help minimize risks regarding the decreased need for a transfusion. State-of-the-art technology and advanced surgical techniques help reduce the volume of potential blood loss while speeding up the surgical procedure. More in depth details of this will be provided to you by your surgeon.

• Pain management for your child, which will be discussed prior to the time of surgery. The concept of pain management in children has changed dramatically in the last twenty years. In the past, children were often left in pain, with the concept that most of them do not remember pain, or that infants have underdeveloped pain pathways and thus do not feel pain. These myths were shown to be false, and today, pain management is not only humane in the care of babies and children, but also helps reduce physiological stress. Optimum pain management helps speed up the healing process and reduces the duration of a potentially long-term hospital stay. Your surgeon will discuss this topic with you and provide further details, especially if the surgical procedure your child will be having necessitates that post-operative pain management be provided.

How Difficult Is the Hospital Registration and Admission Process?

You'll be given complete specialized instructions regarding hospital registration and admission of your child in plenty of time before the surgery is to take place. Your instructions will be specific to the type of procedure your child will be having—ambulatory (same day surgery, where your child will not stay overnight in the hospital) or inpatient (your child will be staying in the hospital for one or more nights). Each hospital and surgery center has its own procedure for the pediatric admission process.

Some facilities provide pamphlets; others allow in-person

orientation tours for parents and children, to help allay anxiety and improve familiarity of the facility. The facilities that perform pediatric surgical procedures on a regular basis and specialize in this area are better equipped and more comfortable in the process of healthcare involving children. If possible, it would be wise for you and your child to make the most of this information regardless how minor you may believe the surgical procedure may be. An in-person visit will be extremely beneficial for both of you.

Will My Child Have to Fast Before Surgery?

Your surgeon may provide specific instructions on food and liquid intake prior to surgery. Restrictions of food and liquids will depend on age of the child. Although general guidelines call for an empty stomach to protect the lungs from accidental reflux of stomach contents, extremely young children are unable to tolerate being without liquids for prolonged periods of time.

Current surgical guidelines call for infants to stop feedings four hours prior to scheduled surgery; however, they can continue with small amounts of clear, non-pulp-containing fluids (e.g., apple juice) until up to two hours prior to surgery. These guidelines can be applied to infants up to four to six months of age.

Infants do not concentrate urine with their young kidneys and cannot tolerate prolonged periods of fluid deprivation. This is not as much of an issue in older children, for whom solids should be stopped six hours prior to the procedure. Clear liquids can be continued until up to three to four hours prior to the procedure. For the safety of your child, please confirm and follow all feeding and fluid intake guidelines that the surgeon instructs you to follow.

Chapter 3
Your Child

How Is It Possible—
Why Does My Baby Need Surgery?

The Developmental Years

During the early years of a child's life, or even before he or she is born, the body is developing, bones are growing, organs are maturing, and body activity is beginning. It is during this time in a child's life that defects within his or her body that were not noticeable before may begin to become apparent. Some defects can be noticed prior to birth by ultrasound, which can potentially detect defects in the heart, lungs, abdomen or head.

In a few cases, depending on the nature of the defect, surgery can be performed in utero (within the uterus), before the child is born. If that isn't possible, plans may be made by your child's physician to schedule the surgery at a specific time soon after the birth. This type of surgery is usually of a more serious nature and may have to be performed in a specific hospital, by a surgeon or surgical team that is highly specialized in that area.

Common Types of Pediatric Surgery

There are other less serious types of surgery that may be necessary during the early developmental years, such as:

- Hernia repair. A hernia is a protrusion of an organ or other structure through the wall that normally contains it. The hole in the wall has to be repaired so that the protrusion is once again contained.

- Tonsillectomy or appendectomy. Whereas once, these surgeries required several days of hospitalization, today, they call for barely more than eight hours in the hospital.

- Trauma. As children become more and more active in sports or other activities, they may fall and injure themselves; facial cuts may require stitches, or broken bones may require surgery.

- Miscellaneous. Illnesses may develop that necessitate surgical procedures.

There are many reasons why your child may need surgery during the early developmental years of life, and maintaining a schedule of regular office visits for your child with the pediatrician is an essential part of monitoring evolving issues.

Chapter 4

. Your Child's Pediatrician

Are Regular Visits to the Pediatrician Important?

Building a Relationship Between Your Child and the Pediatrician

Regular pediatrician visits for your child will help ensure that any developing problems are detected early. During these regular appointments, the physician will examine your child and be watchful for new issues that may have developed since the last office visit. Regular visits will also allow the pediatrician to become familiar with your child's behavior, including subtle changes in the way the child walks, or changes in speech or attentiveness. Each one of us is unique, with mannerisms and traits that belong only to us. Your child's physician will become familiar with these traits and begin to know your child better and better as he or she grows.

In medicine, this is known as a baseline. Just as your physician maintains a baseline for you, the pediatrician maintains one for your child. During your regular visits, the pediatrician will always look at your child against his or her baseline. By examining your child in this way, the pediatrician will be able to notice very subtle changes that might not otherwise be apparent.

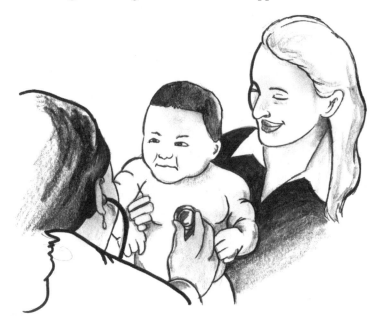

Subtle Changes in Growth and Development

Sometimes, changes are so subtle that we, as parents, may not notice them in the same way a physician would. He or she will also look closely at growth stages in a different way than we would. We may not notice growth changes from day to day, just as we don't notice how much the child has grown until we are shopping for new clothes and see that they need longer pants.

The physician will pay very close attention to growth or changes in specific areas of the body, including:

- Head circumference

- Small abdominal bulges

- Swelling in glands

- Changes in appearance

If the pediatrician does notice an abnormality during the examination, he or she will probably order various tests to confirm that there is a problem. Or, if he or she thinks surgery may be necessary, your child will be referred to a surgical specialist, who will evaluate the abnormality further and recommend the best course of action and remedy. If surgery is recommended, you will want to thoroughly research the best surgeon and the best medical facility for you and your child.

Chapter 5
Finding the Right Surgeon and the Right Place

How Do I Begin the Search?

Who Should I Ask for a Recommendation?

When you first receive the news that your child will need surgery, you will need to sort out several things before you move forward with scheduling the procedure. If the surgery is an emergency, you will probably not have the time to review the following list in detail; if the surgery is not an emergency, there are several steps you can take to find the best surgeon and facility for your child:

1. Ask your child's pediatrician to recommend a surgeon

who has skill and extensive experience in the type
of surgery your child will need.

2. Take the time to visit the healthcare facility, to
make sure that it is child-friendly and can address your
child's needs, as well as your own.

3. Don't hesitate to ask friends and family for
recommendations of surgeons they may have used or
know of through their acquaintances.

4. Email or call the medical board of your state and ask
about the information they have on each licensed
healthcare professional and facility in your area.

5. Check with your insurance company to make sure that
the hospital where your child will have the surgery is
covered under your plan.

6. If you have a computer and access to the Internet, you
can research your local area for specialists. Enter the
medical specialty of the physician you are looking for
and your town's name in Google, or another search
engine. You can also check medical review Websites.
A list has been provided to you in the Resources page 155.

7. Call your local newspaper, radio or TV station and ask
if they have any type of review system for healthcare
providers.

8. Contact the Department of Health in your town and

state and ask if they have listings of physicians in the medical specialty you need. You can also ask about the healthcare facility you will be using for your child.

9. Check with your insurance company to make sure that the surgeon you've selected participates in your plan. If the surgeon does not participate, ask what it might cost for you to use the surgeon anyway—some plans allow you to go out of network, but with an additional cost to you.

Make sure to schedule a consultation appointment with the surgeon you have chosen. During that meeting, you can ask any additional questions you might have and finalize your plans to move forward with the surgery.

Is a Second Opinion Necessary?

The more knowledgeable you are about your child's condition, the better you will be able manage his or her care. Regardless of your surgeon's opinion, if you feel uncertain, do not hesitate to ask questions for further clarification. If you have any doubts—and some insurance companies may insist, in certain cases—it would not hurt to have a second opinion from another surgeon.

Important for You to Know

There may be a limit to how much information the state or local medical review department is legally able to provide, but it's worth checking anyway. Just keep in mind that the flood of lawsuits in our society can be very misleading, and even a medical board's information is often not a good indication of a physician's ability to deliver excellent medical care. Therefore, it is necessary that you contact more than one source when looking for information about physicians.

Finding the Proper Specialist for Your Child

Please make every effort to see an appropriate surgeon—one who is specialized in the type of care your child needs. You should no sooner see a foot doctor for plastic surgery than send a child to surgeon who does not specialize in the type of care that the child needs.

Some areas of this country are not privileged enough to have specialists and super-specialists. Conversely, some metropolitan areas are teeming with pediatric gastroenterologists, pediatric orthopedists, pediatric cardiac surgeons, pediatric neurosurgeons, pediatric otorhinolaryngologists, and many other pediatric surgery specialties.

It is very important that you look for a surgeon with the type of training that your child's procedure will require, as well as a good volume of procedures under his or her belt. It is not so important that he or she graduated from an exclusive college. The more familiar a surgeon is with the needs of your child, the better the chances of a positive outcome.

Find out in advance what type of facility your child will have to be in for the procedure. Research what options are available, as not all towns have the privilege of having a facility that specializes in children's healthcare.

If you have a choice between a medical center that specializes pediatrics and one that does not, go with the one that specializes in care for children. Be assured that at the facility, and its physicians, perform more procedures and are more familiar with circumstances that surround children.

What If It's an Emergency?

Will I Be Able to Select the Surgeon for My Child?

Previously in this book, I touched lightly on the topic of picking the right surgeon and location, but how can you really go about finding the right surgeon now that your child needs surgery? The trail starts either in the pediatrician's office or in the emergency department (ED).

Your options when choosing a physician may be limited if it is your child's misfortune to be brought to the ED. Unless, by divine intervention or privileged influence of knowing about a preferred medical center in advance, your child will be taken to the ED at the closest hospital. This is appropriate during a true emergency, when every second can count.

The Wait in the Emergency Department— How Long Is Too Long?

Most EDs are crowded and depending on the circumstances, the time of day, and the problem at hand, the wait time could be short, or it could be an eternity. It is incredibly important to be patient and supportive with your child during this time, as the stress for both of you will probably be major. In the majority of instances, the triage nurse is very tuned into the most intricate aspects of the wait time for patients, and all efforts are made to shorten the wait time for any child.

There are times, though, when the triage nurse may not realize the urgency of the matter from your perspective, as she is probably very busy. And, if it is a trauma center, the arriving injuries are probably life-threatening. Thankfully, this does not happen often, but it does happen on a very rare occasion.

This actually happened to me, one time when I drove my then infant son to a rural hospital after he was bitten on the head by a family dog. The triage nurse placed us on a waiting list. As a physician, I try not to pull clout, as it is just not a fair way to obtain treatment. However, after waiting fifteen minutes and watching the towel I had wrapped around my son's head become soaked with blood, my patience as a parent wore thin, and my concern as a physician kicked in. In a gentle but firm manner, I made myself heard, and our wait time was eliminated.

If you are faced with this type of situation in the ED, do not hesitate to ask for help again if the status of your child is getting worse. I am not stating this to encourage a constant stream to the triage desk, to try to gain passage through the gauntlet of the ED's stretcher mayhem. Again, this type of situation is rare, and each individual's needs are usually evaluated on a case-by-case basis.

When your child is evaluated by the ED physician, you will be told if a surgical intervention needs to be performed immediately. If your child needs surgery, a surgeon of the appropriate specialty will be consulted. Please, listen carefully to what is going on and what is being said. Take notes if you can and ask questions if the medical jargon is beyond comprehension, or if explanations are contradictory between consulting physicians or other healthcare providers.

Surgical Problems in the Emergency Department—Urgent or Non-urgent

There are two kinds of surgical problems that arise in the ED: those that need immediate intervention, and those that can wait a few days or weeks for an intervention to take place. For example, acute appendicitis is a true emergency and needs to be operated on in a timely fashion. Depending on the circumstances, appendicitis can be treated by antibiotics, but protocol can vary from region to region and from hospital to hospital, as technology changes and as insurance companies begin to rule on different treatment protocols.

In most cases, the on-call surgeon in the hospital will perform the surgery. Unless you are familiar with another surgeon who is affiliated with the hospital, there will be very little choice when it comes to who operates and who performs the anesthesia. There are usually a limited number of surgeons covering the specific specialty that needs to be addressed in the ED. In the majority of cases, there is only one, and that person may not be available in the hospital depending, on the specialty.

In most circumstances, be assured that you are in the hands of very competent healthcare professionals. The vast majority of them have gone into the field of medicine for the purpose of helping others, and that generally shines through. However, circumstances do vary, and situations do change from hospital to hospital. If your child's surgery is not an emergency, and you have time to research the facility, it is important for you to know the policies and the manner in which the hospital you are interested in functions. Will the staff provide attentive care to your child? It's fair to assume that the more educated you become in the process, the better care your child will receive.

Look at the consulting physicians: Do they seem like they've done this on a regular basis, or do they look like deer caught in the headlights of a car? Experienced surgeons are calm and exude confidence, and are deliberate in their actions. They answer questions thoroughly, with no uncertainty, and ask you appropriate questions.

Experienced surgeons know their specialties inside and out and will explain the surgical risks to you; do not misinterpret the risks as uncertainty. The business of life provides no guarantees, but knowing the risks and other dangers that may lurk in the unknown ahead of time will make it easier for you to accept the surgery.

Urgent Surgery—Being Comfortable With Your Child's Surgeon

Once you are given the name of the surgeon in the ED, don't hesitate to find out as much as you can about him or her from the nurses or the ED doctor in charge of your child's care. Every clue will give you confidence in the care of your child. It is very easy to tell, from the manner in which they treat you and your child, whether they have the optimal benefits that you are looking for—the same way you can tell if a waitress at a diner will bring out your meal on time and warm or late and cold.

I like to see healthcare professionals who really enjoy what they're doing. While they may be slightly lackluster at three in the morning, the spark and the caring should shine through. If that is the type of individual that is managing the care of your child, you are in luck.

On the other hand, if the proposed surgeon impresses you

as someone who is not confident in what he or she is doing and could very easily get lost trying to leave the hospital, you should discuss matters with your ED doctor, even though he or she called in the surgeon for consultation. Physicians are human, too.

Non-urgent Surgery—Take Time to Find a Surgeon for Your Child

If the emergency is not urgent and your child has been discharged, and will be waiting at home for surgery in a few days or weeks, then you may have time to do some research about the nature of the illness, the type of care that will be necessary, the type of physician who will need to be consulted, and what type of facility at which the surgery needs to be performed. If you have the time, consult your pediatrician, the Internet and the library—all can be good sources to help you find out the specifics of your child's illness, as well as information about the surgeon who will potentially care for your child.

When you leave the ED, place a call to your child's pediatrician, to bring him or her up to speed regarding your child's health. Your pediatrician can make some suggestions as to whom to see, and if they might be available. You can cross-reference the recommended surgeons with your state's Department of Health, to see what their standing may be. The state Department of Health is a single-dimensional database that has some of the information you'll need.

Remember, a listing of a single lawsuit against a physician is not a determining factor in qualifying the individual as a bad doctor. We live in a sue-happy country and it seems that the majority of physicians out there have been sued at least once, including yours truly. The database will not tell you whether or not the suit was legitimate. However, the database will provide you with information that will add to your research.

Do Your Research

You may already have some reputable Internet sites that you refer to from time to time for your child's health. Many large medical centers sponsor frequently asked question (FAQ) sites or other informative services. The more you know, the better care your child will get, and the less likely you will be to get lost in this unfamiliar jungle.

Don't delay in making an appointment with a reputable specialist, as these physicians are very likely to be busy, and their schedules may be crowded. It may be worth traveling some distance to see a specialist and receive sound advice, even if you choose not to follow through with surgery with that individual. Distance, time or other constraints may prevent you from using an out-of-town surgeon, but at least you will have obtained another opinion. Be sure to thank any specialist you meet with for taking the time to consult with you and divulge valuable information. If the consulting specialist you choose is busy and cannot accommodate your child in his or her schedule, then go down the list for the next specialist.

Once you have obtained an appointment, be prompt; physicians sometimes run late, but not always, and if you are not on time, you will push their schedule even further back for the rest of the day. This may not be a good way to meet your physician. Please let the office know if you are running late, if you know in advance.

Speak to the Anesthesiologist

Another thing you may want to do is to call the hospital and get the number of the anesthesiology department. Ask if you can speak with the pediatric anesthesiologist about the implications of the anesthesia that will be used in your child's upcoming surgery. This is a great opportunity to not only find out what may await you and your child on the day of surgery at that particular center, but to find out about your child's anesthesiologist as well. Most pediatric anesthesiologists are extremely knowledgeable and personable.

Speak to the Surgeon

Once you meet with your child's surgeon, you will be able to inquire about the anesthesiologists you have spoken with and ask which the surgeon will be most comfortable with during the procedure. If you are satisfied with the confidence the anesthesiologist has given you, and you are comfortable with his or her scope of knowledge and caring ability, then you may request this anesthesiologist to take care of your child. You may request this either through your surgeon or by asking the anesthesiologist him- or herself how to request that he or she care for your child.

Once you have developed confidence with the medical team and facility, your child will sense your level of comfort. You will be able to express your support and love much more comfortably because your mind will not be preoccupied with as much uncertainty.

Review the Hospital Services

Be sure to inquire at your chosen facility about what services and amenities they provide to ensure care is specifically directed to children. Once again, the Internet is a great tool for researching and learning about the healthcare providers that will be giving essential care to your child. You may not locate all the information you're looking for on the Internet, but you will be able to gather a great amount that should be helpful to you. Please take into account the Internet source you are using, however; the more reputable the source, the better the information.

Section II
PREPARING FOR SURGERY

Chapter 6
First Steps

How Soon Must the Surgery Be Performed?

Making Preparations

O nce you have identified the surgeon who will perform your child's surgery and the medical facility where the surgery will take place, preparations for the procedure will begin. Depending on the surgery, it may be delayed for a certain amount of time.

- If the surgery needs to occur immediately, such as correction of a cardiac defect, your child may need to be placed on pre-surgical medications by the hospital surgical team.

- Other types of surgery may require that the child's body develop more and grow further before surgical interference can occur, such as in some orthopedic procedures.

- Other surgeries may only require a watch-and-wait approach, such as in the case of hemangiomas (benign blood tumors), which can get larger, remain the same size or resolve and go away on their own. With hemangiomas, it may be dangerous to operate because of the high risk of bleeding. The risk also depends where the hemangioma is—say, on the skin versus next to certain vital organs. In the latter case, a physician must decide whether the tumor is too dangerous to remain, or whether it may interfere with function in the body. This type of decision making will require very intense consideration before an operation is authorized for a child or an infant.

What Is Important to Know As a Parent?

You Are the Vital Link

During this preparatory stage, before the surgery is to be performed, you, the parent, are the vital link between the surgeon and the patient. The physicians rely on you to manage the medical team; maintain calmness and offer support; ensure cooperation between family members and caregivers; oversee and organize consultations, evaluations, laboratory reports, and other medical records; and ensure that all procedure steps are followed.

Wow, this sounds like a lot of work and a lot of responsibility, doesn't it? Yes, and it absolutely is. You are the one who now oversees all of the elements that are essential for the medical team to optimally care for your child.

What Your Child's Physician Wants You to Know

Understand the Procedures

It is not a common occurrence, but on occasion, a parent may fail to follow protocol or proper procedures set by the physician, the hospital, the surgical center or the consulting specialist. This situation will probably increase the stress level of the entire process.

I have seen a few instances wherein parents assume that rules do not apply to them because they are going on vacation and feel the need to change the process to fit their needs. In their opinion, the system will need to understand if certain tests are not done, or if certain consultations are missed. We in the healthcare profession are held to the highest standard and cannot afford to take anything for granted, should anything happen for a variety of reasons. We need the fullest cooperation and assistance of the parents to provide the best care possible.

I have found that most parents will follow every instruction to the letter, although an occasional parent will miss a few steps in between and place tremendous and unnecessary stress on the system. Honest presentation of history and what has been done in the process of care for the child can help the professionals provide care while minimizing the chances of missing anything vital. Sometimes, this does not happen, particularly if there are upset parents or an upset surgical team.

Depending on the type of abnormality or condition that needs to be repaired, the number of visits with the pediatrician, surgeon or other specialist may vary. The child will be seen weeks or days prior to the surgery for final evaluation, which gives the medical team a final opportunity to discuss benefits, options, and pre-operative and post-operative instructions. Medications may need to be added or altered to enhance an optimum surgical outcome. If at any time you feel uncertain about the instructions or what is expected of you on your child's behalf, please do not hesitate to ask.

Chapter 7
The Medical Team

The Anesthesiologist

Once you select your surgeon, you need to line up the next important person in your child's care: the anesthesiologist. Not everyone is familiar with this individual's vital role. More than a "sleep master," the anesthesiologist's role is to keep the patient pain-free, comfortable and alive during surgery. The anesthesia needs of a very young child are different from those of an adult; therefore, a pediatric anesthesiologist should be available, for your child's safety.

Beside the goofy-colored hats and funky gizmos hanging on their belts, pediatric anesthesiologists are passionate physicians who are specially trained to take care of children. You will usually be provided with an anesthesiologist for your child's care by the hospital or surgical center, but you do have options. Not every center has access to a pediatric anesthesiologist. Work with your surgeon to arrange for anesthesia services that will be appropriate for your child.

Parents can greatly help their child anticipate what to expect and allay any anxiety by being loving and supportive. You can openly discuss, in an age-appropriate manner, the medical issue at hand and the manner in which it will be fixed. Please, be patient and supportive throughout the process, and keep these tips in mind:

- Infants up to the age of six months show very little awareness and you do not need to treat them any differently prior to surgery. Just be normally loving toward and supportive with them.

- Children from six months to two years of age have already developed awareness. They can be distracted and entertained easily until the moment of the procedure because of their curious stage.

- Although children up to the age of four may not recall most events, it is important to ensure that the experience is minimally traumatic, to prevent prolonged or life-altering impressions that could impact them forever. Distract young children by playing games with them and showing support and encouragement. In this way, you can help place a positive spin on the experience.

Your Child Needs Your Support— We Need Your Support

Your support, along with the assistance of the operating room staff, will make the events pass quickly. Children up to the ages of six or seven can be very apprehensive and fearful. Your attitude is very important here and by being positive and supportive, you will be extremely helpful in getting them through this rough stage. Trust and faith are key components. Parents on occasion can exaggerate or mislead with good intentions. Do not make promises that you cannot keep.

Easing Your Child's Anxiety Through Assurance

Try to refrain from telling your child that needles will not hurt, as they sometimes do. If you mislead them, they may not believe or trust you in similar circumstances in the future. You can role play with your child, using a doll or a stuffed animal as a patient. You may receive more insight into what your child's expectations are by placing him or her in the role of a doctor or a nurse, and seeing how he or she interacts with the doll.

Your child may pretend that the doll is having the same surgery as he or she is, and may bring the doll to the hospital on the day of surgery so that they can keep each other company throughout the hospital stay. On the day of the surgery, it is helpful to distract your child by playing games or engaging him or her in non-pertinent conversation, to keep him or her as calm as possible. Toward this end, many hospitals have separate waiting areas for children who are going in for surgery, complete with a variety of toys and storybooks.

Managing Your Own Anxiety

Remember, the mood and emotional state of a parent is easily reflected in his or her child. A child of an extremely anxious parent will likely appear anxious and frightened. Parents who are capable of managing their emotional states well often have children who are not very anxious.

The medical environment, as well as the mood and manner of the healthcare professionals, plays a role in the reaction of the child, too. Parents can help mediate the mood immensely because a child will look to his or her parents for clues as to how to behave in the uncertain environment.

Orientation tours for both parents and child have been found helpful in allaying some pre-surgical anxiety. Often, when a parent and child see the surroundings of the medical center and meet the personnel before the actual day of the procedure, they feel much more at ease on day itself, because they have already seen and spoken with many of the staff members.

Multiple Specialists

Parents Can Help With Communication

Certain conditions may require healthcare providers from multiple specialties to coordinate efforts. On rare occasions, this coordination will become complex, requiring some effort by the parents as well, to ensure that all the current information, medical records, insurance and notes are available in a timely manner for the physicians to review prior to the surgery.

Office and Facility Staff

Understanding and Cooperation—Positive Results

Not all physicians' and medical care providers' offices are created with equal efficiency and accuracy, regardless of how capable the physicians may be. If the office staff seems a bit lackluster, it's not a reflection on the virtues of your child's physician; the staff is not always bound by the same standards of service as your physician. Just be kind and cooperative, and ensure that the best interests of your child are met. Walk out of the office being admired by the staff as the most caring and loving parent a child could have. The more liked you are by the office staff, the more fulfilled service and timely care you will receive.

Chapter 8
What the Surgeon Has to Know Before Surgery

Necessary Screening Tests

Patience and Reassurance Throughout the Preparatory Phase

Due to the current trend of hospital cost-cutting and pressure from insurance companies, many hospitals have shifted their emphasis of care. Fewer and fewer patients are admitted into hospitals one or more days prior to their procedures, and workups or preparations for surgery are often done on an ambulatory (walk-in) basis. Preparations for surgery may include X-rays, blood tests and a variety of other evaluations done by medical specialists, depending on the condition that needs to be corrected.

All of this can be very trying for parents and children as they move from appointment to appointment, and from test to test. Waiting times are often long and preparations for tests are often demanding. Please, try to take one day at a time, and be reassuring to your child as you work your way through the preparatory phase.

Instructions for the preparations for specific procedures will be provided by your surgeon's or pediatrician's office. Often, these instructions are customized for the type of procedure, and for your child's health status. For the best outcome, it is crucial that you and your child follow these instructions completely.

It's never a good idea to perform unnecessary blood tests, considering that most children are horrified of needles, and that the entire process leaves them frightened and anxious about the upcoming procedure. Sometimes, this fear can be avoided in healthy children who are scheduled to undergo minor procedures that involve little or no potential blood loss. If that is the case, it is important to determine in advance how much blood loss a child will safely tolerate, and what steps need to be taken to safeguard this.

What Blood Tests Will Be Done?

It is usually important for the surgeon and anesthesiologist to know what the CBC (complete blood count) of the child is before beginning the procedure. If necessary, depending on the blood test results, the surgeon or anesthesiologist will discuss with you the potential needs that may occur during surgery.

There are other blood tests that are not normally ordered except in children with different health considerations—such as certain metabolic problems—or in the case of surgical procedures that could potentially change the blood chemistry through fluid administration or blood or bodily fluid loss. Such children need to have their blood chemistry closely evaluated.

Examples of additional blood chemistry evaluations include tests for sodium, potassium, chloride and glucose, among other elements and compounds. Blood samples may need to be collected two or more times to determine if there is significant change in the blood chemistry, and if that change needs to be medically addressed during and after the surgical procedure.

Will the Blood Tests Hurt?

When appropriate, if blood needs to be drawn, the medical facility may offer to apply a topical ointment or cream with a local anesthetic to the child's hand or arm, to numb the skin. This may take anywhere from thirty to forty-five minutes to take effect. This option is not always available, so it might be helpful to ask in advance if you think you may want this for your child. Remember, the easier the process, the more cooperative the child will be, and the less taxing the experience will be for both parents and healthcare providers.

On occasion, parents may be able to obtain this type of topical anesthetic ointment themselves, and apply it to the area on the child's arm prior to leaving the house before the procedure. The area will have to be protected with a bio-occlusive dressing, which is sold in many pharmacies. This may help save time, and may reduce the impatience and anxiety of the child, rather than waiting in a blood-drawing center for the local anesthetic it provides to work. Please ensure that this is appropriate by asking your child's physician and the blood-drawing center in advance.

Chapter 9
Pre-surgery Procedures

Important to Know in Advance of Scheduled Surgery

Same Day Surgery—How Do I Prepare My Child?

With the increase in ambulatory and same day admission procedures, you are likely to be sent home with a preparation kit from your child's surgeon. This preparation kit and medications will need to be purchased from a pharmacy. Bacteriostatic soap may be one component used during preparation, to cleanse the skin and hair prior to the procedure.

It would be up to your surgeon, and would depend on the type of surgical procedure, if your child would need to be admitted one or more days prior to the operation for specialized testing and preparations. For example, this may happen in the case if a hormone-producing tumor, the effects of which would need to be controlled aggressively, to permit safe removal. This might also happen if there is an infectious component that needs to be treated beforehand, or a hematologic (blood-related) condition that needs close monitoring or management. A variety of circumstances could require early admission; if this is required of your child, your physician will discuss the reasons with you in detail.

Must-haves on the Day of Surgery

It is probably a good idea to bring the following information with you on the day of the procedure. You cannot be sure that all of this information is in the surgical chart already, as it should be. The only way to ensure that everything is there is for you is to bring it with you.

- Information about allergies and any undesirable reactions to medications in the past.

- A list of medications (over-the-counter or prescription) taken in past forty-eight hours.

- A list of medications (over-the-counter or prescription) taken on a regular basis.

- Information about medical problems your child has been treated for, past and present.

- Information about past surgical procedures your child has had.

• Information about problems or complications with surgical procedures, anesthesia or medications in your child's past.

Know the Food and Fluid Restrictions Well in Advance of Surgery

Food and fluid intake varies depending on the age of the child, the procedure type and the policies of the surgical center, and are dictated by the anesthesiologists responsible for the care of your child. The procedure is based on providing a safe environment, and ensures that the child's stomach will be as empty as possible, to prevent regurgitation of stomach contents. The fuller the stomach, the greater the risk of regurgitation; its passage down the windpipe and into the lungs is known as "aspiration." This increases the risk of a serious condition known as "aspiration pneumonitis," which can be deadly for your child. However, this is not much of a concern in the case of an infant or child who is fed according to a previously scheduled regiment.

Your surgeon will give you specific instructions regarding the limitations on food and fluid intake for your child, based on the scheduled time of the procedure. Each child is limited as far as the period of time during which they can safely remain without food or fluids, depending on their age. Most surgical centers will limit food, formula and milk intake during the six to eight hours prior to surgery, depending on the age of the child. Water intake will be limited from two to four hours prior to the procedure.

Please, adhere closely to these instructions and do not hesitate to ask any questions or address any concerns you may have. If your child has violated the food or liquid intake guidelines, please make sure to inform your child's healthcare providers immediately. This is for your child's safety. The procedure may not necessarily be cancelled, but it may be delayed until sufficient time has passed and it can be conducted safely.

Chapter 10
Understanding Anesthesia

Addressing Your Concerns

Are You Concerned About Anesthesia for Your Child?

Most parents I have spoken with have expressed to me that anesthesia is their number-one concern when their child is having surgery.

How will their child react to the anesthesia? How dangerous is it? I have already touched upon the implications and impact of anesthesia on a child, but I feel that this topic needs its own section, to thoroughly address as many of your questions and concerns as possible.

I have found, throughout my fifteen-plus years of practicing anesthesia, that most individuals are not familiar with the vital role of the anesthesiologist. My art is a bit of an enigma and a mystery, not only to the non-medical individual but also to most experts in other fields of the medical profession.

In simple terms, my purpose as an anesthesiologist in the operating room is to ensure the complete comfort and absolute safety of the patient while the procedure is being performed. Of course, it is quite a bit more involved than that, but this is the simplest way to look at it.

What Are Anesthetists?

Two types of individuals can administer anesthesia: One is an anesthesiologist and the other is a nurse anesthetist.

• The anesthesiologist is a medical doctor who spends an additional four years after medical school studying anesthesiology. The first year of training is an internship that can be in either pediatrics, internal medicine or surgery. This is a very crucial period of time, during which the anesthesiologist learns the basics of patient care and management. An intern spends an entire year performing so-called "scut work"—running laboratories, transporting patients, drawing blood, and helping nurses perform basic but vital patient-care tasks. He or she performs these tasks under the watchful eye of a fully trained physician instructor. There is always someone else who can do scut work, but this is the best way for a physician not only to understand the inner workings of patient care, but to develop basic skills in obtaining information from patients that is crucial to their care, and examining them and developing diagnostic and treatment skills. After the internship, three years are spent in the operating room, learning the ins and outs of anesthesia. At the completion of a residency program, an anesthesiologist may choose to spend another one or two years further refining his or her skills in a program that specializes in pediatric anesthesia. The American Board of Anesthesia (ABA) regulates and governs this entire process rigorously by ensuring that its members have not only fulfilled the necessary requirements, but have passed the rigorous examination process to be board-certified by the ABA.

- The certified registered nurse anesthetist (CRNA) devotes two additional years, on top of his or her nursing education, to become a nurse anesthetist. These nurses work in conjunction with anesthesiologists to perform crucial duties in caring for patients in hospitals. In certain private surgical centers, they may work with out the involvement of an anesthesiologist, under the supervision of the operating surgeon. Nurse anesthetists play a crucial role in regions where there are shortages of anesthesiologists.

The anesthesiologist who will play a major role in caring for your child has undoubtedly devoted years of studying and training to the understanding of anatomy, physiology (the way the body and its organs work) and pharmacology (the way medications work, and how they interact with each other and with organs of the body). There is no way that I can possibly list all the fine details of what is involved in the training process without taking up too much valuable space in this book, and probably putting you to sleep in the process.

Understanding what is involved in the medical training of the anesthesiologist and the certified nurse anesthetist may help you appreciate their competence; it may comfort you to know that your child is in the best of hands. An anesthesiologist is usually assigned to a specific operating room for an entire day, covering whatever procedures take place in that one room, but you can request to have a specific anesthesiologist care for your child, even if he or she is not originally scheduled to be in your OR.

Are There Risks Associated With Anesthesia?

For most healthy children, the risk of anesthesia is very little. In children over the age of six months, the risk is similar to an adult.

With children, however, many of the instruments used to perform the anesthetic are smaller, and doses of the medications are lower depending on the age and size of the child. As I mentioned earlier, it takes a combined effort of parents and healthcare providers to adequately educate and encourage the child through the process prior to drifting off to sleep.

It takes approximately six months for internal organs to develop adequately to process the medications necessary for anesthesia. This does not mean that the medications are not processed and eliminated from the body in an infant, or that an infant is in any danger. It's just that their organs are inefficient and because of this, the anesthesiologist, in certain cases, will need to adjust the doses for the needs of the baby.

With an infant, the approach to surgery is that much more delicate because of the size of the child; a great deal goes into consideration when performing surgery on a child that small. However, rest assured that your child's healthcare professionals will work as a team to ensure that the procedure goes as smoothly as possible, and that the small child is kept extremely safe.

When you are handing your child off to an anesthesiologist, be assured that this individual has put a great deal of consideration into the well-being of your child, and will make your child the most important person in his or her life while under his or her care.

What the Anesthesiologist Wants You to Know

From my own personal standpoint as an anesthesiologist, I would like to recommend that you and your child meet or speak with the anesthesia care provider in advance of the surgery. This will help build a rapport and make a connection, so that you and your child can be confident and comfortable with the person who will be in charge of your child's life.

When I find out that I will be caring for a child, I contact the parents in advance, to give them an idea of what is expected of them, what they can expect from me, and what they should anticipate before, during and after their child's surgery. This communication also offers a great opportunity for me to introduce myself as the attending anesthesiologist and help the parents feel comfortable.

I have experienced both ends of the spectrum, from parents who were knowledgeable and comfortable with the way things should be going, to parents who seemed as though they had no idea of what was happening and appeared uncomfortable with the situation, the healthcare providers and even themselves.

Parents have always played a vital role in helping me make the care of their child go smoother, by facilitating and easing the process. On the other hand, I also realize that parents can compound issues as well. If the parents feel comfortable, they will be assuring with their child, thus reducing, if not eliminating, the awkwardness of the situation. I believe that if I have a chance to speak with the parents briefly before the procedure and familiarize them with what to expect, the process will definitely be smoother, and less stressful for both parents and child.

Not all medical centers or anesthesiologists follow this type of protocol. I suggest that you inquire with your surgeon's office about speaking with your anesthesiologist in advance of the procedure.

An Interesting Case Study

Throughout my medical career, I have experienced many challenging and rewarding circumstances. One of the most rewarding experience resulted from a situation wherein the parents of a seven-year-old patient were from a foreign country and spoke limited English. The child was having a surgical procedure very similar to another he'd had previously, in his country of origin.

The mother had difficulty comprehending the great discrepancy in how her child was to be treated here. Her first concern was that we were planning to do the procedure in a private operating room in the oral surgeon's office, rather than in a very large hospital. She could not understand why her child was not staying in the hospital for the procedure and remaining overnight. What if something happened? What was going to happen to her child? The questions were realistic and numerous, and I realized that if she was not able to understand the reasons why the procedure would be performed as planned, her discomfort would translate into a series of awkward and unhappy moments long before we reached the operating suite.

I spoke with her twice before the procedure, once a month in advance. As a rule, my usual conversations with parents and patients do not last more than fifteen minutes. Because of the language barrier, however, I needed about forty-five minutes to help her understand the differences in culture and the standard of healthcare between her country and ours.

Here in the United States, insurance companies have been a great force in shaping, influencing and impacting the standard of healthcare. They have been profoundly instrumental in establishing why many of our procedures have become ambulatory in nature—because they are in the business of saving healthcare dollars.

What Are the Different Types of Anesthesia?

For most children who require surgery, the most common format of anesthesia is general anesthesia. If children are not able to cooperate in the placement of an intravenous line for medication delivery, which is usually the case with children younger than seven years of age, a clear plastic mask is placed over the nose and mouth to administer the medication that will help the child drift off to sleep. Some anesthesiologists "flavor" the masks with a fruit or gum aroma so that smell of plastic and medical gases are not too offensive.

There are four stages of anesthesia as the child begins to drift off to sleep.

- In the first stage, when the mask is initially applied, the child may appear sedated.

- The second stage is also known as the "excitatory" stage. As the child begins to feel the effects of the anesthesia, the nervous system may behave involuntarily because of the temporary imbalance of the neural pathways. To put it simply, the child may experience involuntary movements of the arms and legs while drifting off to sleep. To the untrained eye, it may seem as thought the child is fighting against the anesthetic. With many new anesthetics, this phenomenon is very quick and often passes before anyone realizes that there had been some form of excitement. I need to mention this because parents may become unnecessarily upset if they witness their child struggling.

• The third stage is the perfect stage for surgery. This is a broad stage identified by relaxation of the muscles, and steadying of the heart rate and blood pressure. The breathing can vary from slow, regular and spontaneous to complete cessation and needing assistance. In this stage, there is complete sensory loss, and surgery can commence without the patient being aware of it.

• The fourth stage is characterized by overdosage. Dangers of respiratory and cardiac arrest are imminent.

General Anesthesia

General anesthesia, done by mask or intravenously, is the most common way in which a child is anesthetized for surgery. Through this means, the child will be unconscious and unable to feel anything while the surgery is performed.

It is important for parents to know that all aspects of the child are closely monitored during the procedure, including:

• Depth of anesthesia

- Oxygen level in the child's body

- Heart rate

- Heart rhythm

- Blood pressure

- Temperature

- Body position

- Exhaled gases, when the breathing is controlled with a ventilator

- Many other factors, depending the type and extent of procedure

Local Anesthesia

Some surgeons may elect to inject local anesthesia into the wound after the child is asleep, either prior to surgery or near the end of the procedure. Such an injection may help reduce the depth of general anesthesia, if the surgery is fairly superficial and not impacting major internal organs. It also helps reduce some of the blood loss in the superficial layers of the skin, and allows the surgeon to work more efficiently because he or she spends less time dabbing the wound to improve visualization.

Some formulations of local anesthetics contain adrenaline, which can reduce blood loss and help the numbing effects of the local anesthetics to last longer. Because of this, the surgeon will elect to inject a little bit of local anesthesia into the wound at the end of the procedure, to help pain relief last a little longer.

Another method of using local anesthetics is known as "regional anesthesia techniques." These techniques are designed to block or numb a group of nerves that provide sensation to certain regions or parts of the body. These will vary depending on the age of the child and the location of the procedure. There are different types of regional anesthetic techniques; your surgeon and anesthesiologist will discuss them in more detail with you, if applicable.

Types of Regional Anesthesia

- Caudal blocks—used in procedures on the lower extremities or lower abdomen. The term *cauda* is Latin, and refers to a tail. A caudal block is administered after the child is asleep. He or she is turned to the side, and the skin over the lower back is sterilized with alcohol or antimicrobial soap. An injection is made near the tailbone (also known as the "coccyx"). In this area, there are two well-defined bones with an empty space between them. The space is contiguous with the space that contains the nerves from the spinal cord. This space can be accessed safely with no risk of coming into contact with the nerves, which are further up the spine—though enough local anesthetic can be injected to reach and numb them. An anesthesiologist can lengthen the duration of pain relief following the procedure by performing the caudal near the end of surgery. With age, this empty space becomes less defined and is not as easily accessible, and we need to resort to other regional anesthetic techniques, like spinals and epidurals, to achieve the same effect. One important fact that most people are not aware of is that the spinal cord stops growing after birth—it remains the same size. Thus, the nerves coming off the spinal cord need to stretch to reach the lower part of the spinal column as we age and grow taller.

• Epidural blocks—very similar to caudals in the way they are performed. Epidurals are placed in children requiring extensive surgical procedures involving the lower extremities or abdomen. Only patients who will remain in the hospital for more than one night can benefit from the long-use effects of an epidural. An epidural provides pain relief through a very thin, plastic catheter that is inserted in the epidural space in the small of the back. The epidural space is a very narrow area surrounding the spinal canal. When local anesthesia is injected into this space, it numbs the nerves that provide sensation to the abdomen and lower extremities. For very young children and babies, the caudal space, described above, can be used to place a catheter up into the epidural space because the spaces are contiguous.

• Spinal blocks—work the same way as epidurals. A very thin needle is utilized to deposit a very small amount of local anesthetic in the fluid that bathes the spinal cord and the nerves that emerge from the spinal cord. Unlike the epidural, there is usually no catheter left in to further inject more medications. Instead, enough medication is placed to last the duration of the surgical procedure— anywhere from one to three hours, depending on the type of medication used. Currently, a great many hernia repairs are performed on premature babies under spinal anesthesia, to help reduce the incidence and risk of apnea, or a stoppage of breathing, which can be associated with general anesthesia immediately following surgery, and until the anesthetic has completely worn off.

- Nerve blocks—injections that specifically numb major nerve branches that provide sensation to the arms or legs. This technique is commonly performed in older children, usually in hospitals that specialize in orthopedic surgical procedures. If the child is mature enough to cooperate and agree, and the parents are willing to consent, then the child will be sedated, and the area where the block will be administered will be cleaned with alcohol or antimicrobial soap. The skin will be numbed with an injection from a very thin needle; then, the nerves will be numbed using specialized needles for the nerve block. In a nerve block, local anesthesia is injected into the area surrounding the nerves. The local anesthetic bathes the nerves and numbs them. This helps reduce the amount of anesthesia needed to keep the patient asleep while the surgery is being performed. In this day and age, specially modified ultrasound techniques are used to place the local anesthetic in very close proximity of the nerves. Regional anesthetic techniques contribute to faster wake-up and prolonged pain relief, and reduce the amount of pain medication needed. Since anesthesiologists perform these techniques frequently in medical centers, they are very comfortable executing them with few difficulties.

It is important to note that all procedures have risks of side effects including infections, bleeding (if a blood vessel is inadvertently struck by the needle) or ineffectiveness, if the local is not placed close enough to the nerve branches. The anesthesiologist will be able to expand on the specifics of these techniques, should they be considered as part of your child's procedure.

Intravenous Sedation

Intravenous sedation is not used often, but can play a role in surgery for older children, along with the types of anesthetics described above. With this form of sedation, medications are administered through an intravenous line, allowing the child to be in a state of sleep while the surgeon performs surgery, with the assistance of local anesthesia. Intravenous sedation can be applied, for example, in surgical procedures performed on the skin, superficial procedures done on the hands or feet, and minor oral surgical procedures.

In many medical centers, this type of anesthesia is frequently used for diagnostic procedures in children, such as MRI, CT scan, endoscopy, spinal tap, bone marrow biopsy, radiation and nuclear medicine therapy for tumors.

Section III
THE ACTUAL OPERATION

Chapter 11
What to Expect

Arriving at the Surgery Center

Be Familiar With Procedures Before You Come

D epending on the type of procedure and/or the health of your child, hospitalization may be required prior to the procedure. However, with most procedures, patients are allowed to come to the facility on the day of the procedure and are discharged the same day, or up to a few days following the surgery.

- Please arrive promptly with your child on the day of the procedure. Surgical schedules often change throughout the day because of cancellations and additions of procedures. On occasion, procedures may be inserted into the schedule and create an unavoidable delay for other scheduled patients. When this happens, the delay can cause tremendous stress for both the patients and the parents. Surgical team members work together to avoid such scenarios, particularly when young children are scheduled for surgery. However, on very rare occasions, this may not be avoidable. If this happens to you and your child, everything will be done to provide care for your child in a timely manner. It would not be inappropriate for you to ask the surgical liaison or someone at the surgical desk about the status of your case, or what steps are being taken to provide care for your child.

• Please dress your child in clothes that are easy to put on and remove. Although surgical dressings will cover the wound, some procedures may result in oozing, and blood may tinge your child's clothes. With tonsillectomies, for example, there can be bloody sputum; with nasal procedures, there can be a bloody drip. Add to this a restless, groggy or uncooperative child, and blood can easily end up on clothes. Children can also experience nausea. Ask your surgeon if you should come prepared for an unplanned experience in this area. Always be prepared with a basin or towels. Because of these potential situations, you should take care in choosing the appropriate clothing for your child. Opt for something that is easy to wear, that will keep him or her warm and dry, and that you might not feel bad about throwing away afterwards. You can also consider bringing an extra set of clothes for your child, in case they are needed.

If your child is having same day surgery (outpatient or ambulatory), it is vital that you follow your physician's instructions carefully. It is most important that you comply with your physician's strict guidelines regarding the restriction of food and fluid intake provided to you by your physician as described in Chapter 9. Also, as discussed above, it is recommended that you arrive promptly at the registration area, as the registration period can sometimes be extensive, and any delay in appearance could result in postponement or cancellation of the procedure.

As I explained in a prior chapter, the surgical schedule is extremely dynamic, and procedures, on occasion, are cancelled or added, for a variety of reasons. If you are unavoidably delayed, please call ahead to inform the surgical center so that the staff can take the necessary steps to change the arrangements for your arrival. But, above all, try to allow plenty of time to arrive at the surgical site on a timely basis.

Upon admission to the surgical facility, your child will receive an identification bracelet with his or her name and chart number on it. Special drug sensitivity and allergy bracelets will also be applied if your child has experienced any type of reaction to medications in the past.

> It is your very important responsibility to ensure that the information on your child's hospital bracelet and the information on your child's chart match the information in his or her medical history.
>
> ALWAYS advise the medical staff involved in the care of your child of ANY and ALL inaccuracies that may appear on your child's identification bracelet.

Please, during this time, do not be alarmed if you are asked the same questions repeatedly. Many questions, especially those pertaining to allergies and sensitivities, will be repeated each time a new healthcare provider becomes involved in the care of your child. This practice helps confirm the information that is already contained in the chart.

Managing the Anxious Time Before Surgery

The anxious moments of anticipation prior to surgery are the most stressful for parents and child. This is true for anyone, at any age, who is awaiting surgery.

To help lessen the stress of the pre-surgery time, some medical centers have tried to create waiting areas with ambiance, offering distractions for the children such as fish tanks, toys and music. These exciting, often wildly painted waiting rooms also provide opportunities for you to meet with your child's anesthesiologist just prior to the procedure, to hear the plan of action.

Meet With the Anesthesiologist Before Surgery

At this time, the anesthesiologist will provide details of expected events and discuss whether or not the surgical team plans to use an intravenous (IV) line or a mask to put the child to sleep.

The anesthesiologist will evaluate the child before the surgery and determine the best course of care. Placement of an intravenous line may not be an option for a screaming, thrashing child or anyone who is under six or seven years of age. For them, a general anesthetics using a mask that delivers oxygen and a high concentration of inhalational anesthetic may be more appropriate.

In some centers, a local anesthetic cream may be applied on the skin where an intravenous line might be anticipated. In other medical centers, the anesthesiologist may elect to give your child a sedative, orally or through other means, prior to taking him or her into the operating room. Each child and circumstance will be evaluated on an individual basis.

Can I Accompany My Child Into Surgery?

Some anesthesiologists allow a parent to accompany his or her child into the operating room. If that happens, it is important that the parent follows all instructions to protect the sterility and integrity of the operating room.

Every facility that allows a parent to participate in the child's induction into anesthesia has its own policies about how such a situation may proceed. The participation may be as minimal as providing your child sips of apple juice, spiked with a sedative, up to an hour prior to the procedure, or as involved as walking your child to the operating room or an ante room, where you may assist your child into sleep. Depending on the preference of the anesthesiologist, you may be allowed to hold your child in your arms while a clear plastic mask is applied to his or her face, and he or she drifts off to sleep. There is no right or wrong format when it comes to this, because an anesthesiologist will evaluate each situation individually and determine the proper way to perform the anesthetic.

If you accompany your child, you will be asked to wear either surgical scrubs or a bunny suit, depending on what the facility provides, with a hat and mask. Please do not attempt to shake hands with individuals who might be scrubbed in the operating room, to greet them or express your gratitude. Also, do not touch instruments or sterile surfaces.

The operating room will appear stark and ominous, but it is your *very important role* to remain calm, loving and supportive of your child while working with the medical personnel to keep your child as calm as possible. If for any reason you feel as if this is overwhelming, and you are having difficulty, please be vocal in expressing yourself. Matters will only become more complex should you faint or lose composure.

If that happens, however, rest assured that an adept anesthesiologist or nursing staff may be able to distract a child sufficiently to accomplish the necessary tasks, after assisting the parent to leave the operating room. All of this may sound like basic information, but under extraordinary circumstances, some individuals become upset and lose a grasp of everything that keeps them balanced. This is certainly understandable for a parent whose child is undergoing a surgical procedure.

Most parents deal with these situations appropriately, but for a few, the circumstances may become a bit much, and they may find themselves unable to control their emotions. An overly emotional parent will not be of any benefit to his or her child, other than adding an additional element of stress in the operating room. All parents are escorted from the operating suite while their children drift off to sleep, and asked to wait in the surgical waiting area for the doctor or surgical representative to join them and provide an update.

Waiting, Waiting, Waiting

Patience Is So Hard

While your child is in surgery, you will be asked to wait in the surgical waiting area. There is no question that this is a very trying time for any parent. Until the surgeon comes out of the operating room and tells you everything is okay, you will certainly be anxious.

Time will move faster if you bring something to read or do. Cell phones are disruptive to other individuals' privacy and usually violate hospital policy, so don't plan on using your phone unless you step outside the hospital. Muted, hand-held video games are okay, however. And, most facilities have a coffee shop or dining area.

If the procedure is taking significantly longer than you expected, don't hesitate to inquire with the operating room liaison or at the operating room desk. I'm not suggesting you make this a habit, however, as each time you inquire about the progress of your child's surgery, the surgeon needs to be distracted, to be informed that a family member needs to know how much longer surgery will take. It is certainly understandable that you, as a waiting parent, will be concerned, but do try to be patient.

What Happens After the Surgery Is Complete?

Once the surgery is complete, the surgeon will immediately step out to have a discussion with the parents. When your child emerges from the anesthesia and is once again breathing on his or her own and opening his or her eyes, he or she will be transported to the post-anesthesia care unit (PACU). Most healthcare facilities will allow one or both parents to visit their child, and to remain with their child once he or she is situated in the recovery room.

When you first see your child after surgery, he or she may appear sedated or restless, or be crying. While in the PACU, each child is continuously evaluated by the PACU physician, the nurse and other staff who personalize their care to fit the needs of each patient. Often, a child may cry not because he or she is in pain, but because of disorientation and fear.

It's not always in the best interest of patients to eliminate all pain immediately after surgery, because pain is sometimes an important indication of internal bleeding—something that physicians must be able to detect immediately. Pain medication might mask the symptoms and can often cause serious side effects, and therefore must be administered delicately and skill-fully in terms of dosage. The requirements vary from patient to patient, as well as from procedure to procedure.

Who Decides When My Child Can Go Home?

When specific criteria are met in the PACU, if your child's surgery was an ambulatory procedure, he or she will be discharged at the discretion of the surgeon or anesthesiologist. They may prolong the hospital stay if they are concerned about your child, and feel as though he or she needs to remain overnight. Please trust your healthcare providers to make the best decision for your child's well-being. Also, please feel free to ask questions if the treatment plans change.

Routinely, the surgeon will meet with you after the surgery, to give you an overview of how the surgery progressed and how he or she anticipates that recovery will proceed. If your surgeon is not immediately available, a nurse or an operating room liaison may be able to convey your concerns to the surgeon, and inform you when that surgeon will be available to address your questions.

Nausea and vomiting can be occasional side effects of general anesthesia, particularly if the surgical procedure involved the head, ear, neck or abdomen. During or after procedures involving the mouth, throat or nasal sinuses, small amounts of bloody fluid may be swallowed or may drain from the location of the surgical site into the stomach, also causing nausea. Modern surgical and anesthetic techniques can reduce the incidence of nausea and vomiting, but they cannot completely eliminate it for everyone. If nausea and vomiting become an issue for your child following surgery, the medical care team will evaluate your child and recommend the best course of action to minimize these side effects.

Always Keep Accurate Records of Incidents

Children grow up and move away from home, and when the time comes for medical care, some of the records in the medical center may be difficult to find. Details often blur and become vague, thus putting your child at risk of treatment problems, or even neglect of treatment.

Healthcare professionals may be uncertain in their attempts to treat unless they know all of the circumstances surrounding the original adverse reactions. I have been told by some patients, "I am allergic to an antibiotic, but I'm not sure which one." This type of vagueness leads to uncertainty and can become a severe issue when an antibiotic is called for in treatment.

Therefore, I urge you to keep accurate records of all undesirable reactions your child may experience, and have it available for physicians and other healthcare professionals at any time it is needed.

What Is an Intravenous Line?

The intravenous (IV) line is an indwelling catheter inserted into a vein through the skin. It is the lifeline through which fluids and medications are safely administered before, during and after surgery. It is also an important vehicle for the administering of medications such as pain relievers and antibiotics. It will remain in place until the physician decides that it is medically safe to remove it. This is usually done immediately before discharge from the hospital.

Parents, please do not be alarmed if your child is brought out of the operating room with excess bandages, drainage tubes, a breathing tube and other paraphernalia. Depending on the duration and complexity of the surgery, the location of the operation on your child's body, and the medical condition that the surgery addressed, each child will present to the PACU in a different manner. The surgeon will most likely have explained all of this to you before the surgery, when you went over what to expect. However, changes may occur during surgery and when this happens, alterations may have to be made in the way the child is treated post-surgery.

In the PACU, fluid is generally given to the patient through an intravenous (IV) line that may be inserted in the arm. The IV site is overseen by a vigilant nurse who applies multiple layers of tape, bandages and arm boards, which are used to secure the IV. All of this is done to immobilize the arm and minimize the risk an accidental removal of the very important IV.

All fluid and medication will be administered through the IV. A child emerging from the stupor of anesthesia may flail, thrash and crash about the recovery bed, leading to a dislodgement of the IV, the only modality by which fluids will be administered until the child regains enough consciousness to take oral fluids, unless otherwise contraindicated by the type of surgical procedure.

Discharge After Same Day Surgery

Questions and Instructions— Don't Be Afraid to Ask Anything

When your child is discharged from the hospital, the nurses in the PACU will provide you with important information to help you take care of your child at home. Please don't hesitate to ask any questions at this time. It is easier to address all questions before you leave the medical center than to try to find the answers later on, when you're already home.

If your child is scheduled to go home on the day the surgery takes place, you will probably notice that the effects of anesthesia last for hours, and possibly for more than a day. The anesthetic agents sometimes linger for more than twenty-four hours in the body. Pain medications can add or enhance the lingering effects of anesthesia as well.

It is very important that you follow the post-operative instructions closely. The instructions will usually include bed rest to minimize the likelihood of bleeding, pain or disruption of the surgical site, and to preclude injuries from falling or other accidents related to the effects of anesthesia.

Things to keep in mind when your child is ready for discharge from the hospital:

- The hospital stay may be prolonged if the surgeon feels that it is necessary

- Nausea and vomiting can occur after general anesthesia

- Keep accurate records of side effects after surgery

- Effects of anesthetic agents can last up to twenty-four hours after surgery

- Follow post-operative instructions closely

If an Overnight Stay or an Extended Stay Is Required

What Can I Bring to My Child's Room?

Certain surgical procedures require overnight or extended stays in the hospital. Should your child need to remain in the hospital for any length of time, please familiarize yourself with all hospital policies, especially those regarding visitation hours and accommodations for parents. Policies vary greatly from hospital to hospital and what is okay for one may not be for another.

Some hospitals are quite strict regarding visiting hours, while other hospitals allow limited accommodations for at least one parent in the child's room at all times. Policies may also vary within the same hospital, between shared and private hospital rooms. If the hospital allows for cots or other accommodations in the child's room, please understand that it is a privilege to be available for your child and as such, it is important that you allow the hospital and nursing staff to tend to their necessary duties.

On occasion, a parent may overlook the fact that his or her child is not be the only patient in the hospital. I have witnessed instances wherein a parent became overwhelmed by circumstances and instead of enhancing the care of his or her child, interfered with the staff's ability to care for everyone.

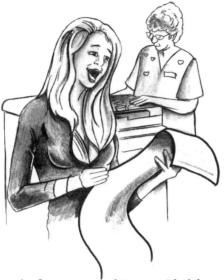

Special Needs for You and Your Child

You may find it helpful to look at the type of amenities the hospital may offer for you and your child and plan in advance to take care of any your special needs. For example, you may need to obtain meals in advance for yourself, or eat in a common eating room or cafeteria, depending on hospital policy.

The hospital staff will definitely appreciate your help in keeping all prohibited objects off of the patient floors. Prohibited items may include cellular phones, food, radios, televisions, compact disc and DVD players, toys, games and other items. These objects may contribute to disruption of care, and interfere with your child's rest, and that of other patients. Every medical institution varies in its policies regarding prohibited items in pediatric care areas; know in advance what can be brought to enhance the comfort and care of your child and what cannot. If you are allowed to bring some of these items, please be aware of your surroundings and be considerate of others sharing the same space.

Dietary Restrictions

Your child's diet will be specified by his or her doctor, and must be strictly adhered to. Please do not take it upon yourself to modify the doctor's dietary instructions.

Occasionally, parents confuse the hospital with another institution that offers room service as an amenity. Remember, patient call buttons should be used for patient care only. The nurses are trained professionals who will do their best to make your child's stay as smooth as possible.

Pain Management After Surgery

It is normal to expect that your child will experience some degree of pain and discomfort after surgery. The nurses will follow the physicians' orders in administering medications to help alleviate discomfort without posing dangerous side effects. Be comforting and supportive of your child while he or she is recovering under the care of the hospital professionals.

Prior to your child's discharge from the hospital, you will be provided with instructions for his or her care once home. Please address your questions to the nursing staff or physician prior to leaving the hospital. If there are questions that the nurse is unable to answer, you may be directed to your child's surgeon.

What You Can Expect After Discharge

Optimally, your child should be returned to a peaceful and safe environment at home, with minimal physical activity, minimal noise and few if any distractions. The most difficult period will be the first twenty-four hours to forty-eight hours following surgery, when the wound is fresh and the swelling the greatest. Follow your surgeon's recommendation for activity level, and ensure that all post-operative instructions are followed exactly as written. This will help ease your child's recover, and speed it along.

As I previously mentioned, too much activity too soon after surgery can cause disruption of your child's wound, bleeding (which can also result from increased blood pressure), or exacerbation of pain and swelling near the surgery site. Rest and comfort will help speed your child's recovery.

If given at higher doses, pain medications may contribute to unpleasant and dangerous side effects, ranging from nausea to the possibility of cessation of breathing. Please, always make sure to very carefully follow the dosing guidelines set by your child's physician. Also, make sure that the information on the medication label matches what your doctor wrote on the prescription. As rare as it may be, sometimes, the wrong prescription can be dispensed.

> *Most importantly, keep all medications out of the reach of all children. Younger children often like to mimic their parents and might not think twice about popping open a pill bottle and swallowing a few of whatever is inside. As difficult as it may be to take care of one child who is recovering, the stress upon any parent would be increased tenfold if they had to worry about another child in the household who has consumed incorrect medications.*

- Support and encourage your recovering child as activity is expanded, under the recommendation of the physician.

- Contact your surgeon if your child's pain level changes and there is a need for medication beyond what has been prescribed. The need for more medication must not be determined independently of the advice of your child's physician; nor should you administer additional medication without first consulting him or her. There may be underlying causes for your child's increased pain, such as internal bleeding or infection, that will require immediate intervention.

• Wound care in the hospital will be managed by the nursing staff, under the direction of the surgeon. This involves keeping the wound and its dressing dry and clean. The physician or nurse caring for your child may show you how to change the dressing, monitor drainage of the surgical incision, and watch for excess bleeding or signs of infection. Please follow these instructions closely and ask questions if the instructions are not clear.
Wound care can vary with the type and location of the incision. For the average incision, the key is to keep the wound clean, dry and free of interference. The surgeon will provide specific instructions on how to care for the wound once the child is discharged from the hospital.

• Most patients need to be seen by the surgeon within a week of discharge, to ensure proper healing. At that time, the surgeon will most likely remove the sutures or surgical staples from the surgical site.

Chapter 12
Risks of Surgery in Children

Unique Challenges for the Surgeon, the Anesthesiologist and the Medical Care Team

M any of the risks children face during surgery are similar to the risks adults face during surgery, especially as far as bleeding and infection are concerned. However, medical advancement and improved knowledge have contributed to making modern surgery the safest in the history of man.

In the past, many children with common surgical issues were not operated on because of limitations in technology. Now, with the advancement of microscopic procedures and other technological and surgical skills, we are able to tackle some of the most challenging medical issues that our children face—even such intricate surgery as the separation of conjoined twins, which can be done successfully depending on the dgree of organ sharing between the children. Unfortunately, while this ability now exists in the United States and other advanced countries, it still does not in some of the third world countries.

Children present a unique set of challenges for surgeons, anesthesiologists and the rest of the medical care team. Their anatomic structures are smaller, the organs closer together, and their ability to tolerate blood loss, in most cases, is less. And, since their body size is smaller, they are more prone to loss of body heat during surgery and in the recovery room.

Monitoring Patients During Surgery

With the development of improved technology and advances in anesthetic techniques, physicians are now able to monitor patients in surgery more closely than ever before. The risk of mortality (death) in healthy patients undergoing simple surgical procedures is extremely low. According to the *Journal of Healthcare Technology*, the number is estimated to be 1 death in 50,000 to 1 death in 100,000.

The risk of surgery decreases as a child's age increases. However, a child's risks during surgery rises if he or she has serious anatomic or medical abnormalities. It is not possible to discuss every risk factor here because of the complexity and rarity of many medical states; in short, it is beyond the scope of this type of guide.

Infants, Aged Three Months and Under

The greatest surgical risk arises in the case of an infant under three months of age. Between birth and three months, a child undergoes many growth changes that help it adapt to life outside of the womb:

- Many organs, including the heart, lungs, liver and kidneys, begin to mature, to allow normal metabolism and function.

- Not only does the circulation of the child undergo a radical change, but so does the child's blood.

- The child emerges from the relatively oxygen-deprived environment of the womb into an oxygen-rich atmosphere outside of the mother.

While this transformation of life is nothing less than a miracle, it does present a unique set of challenges, which will need to be confronted by the surgeon and the anesthesiologist.

Surgeries involving this age group are usually extremely important, and are the results of major developmental defects in the children, involving organs or organ systems. Physicians usually try to delay most surgical procedures for this age group until after the infant has grown past the first three months, if possible.

The infant gradually develops physiologically—over the next year and a half, the organs and body functions become those of a miniature adult. The infant begins to develop awareness after the first six months and from this point on, parents need to take this into consideration, and be nurturing and loving through the most challenging aspect of the child's life. Most healthy children, from the ages of two on, share the same low surgical risks as adults, but their fear and apprehension add another facet that parents must deal with prior to the onset of surgery.

Asthma

Asthma is a medical condition involving the lungs, characterized by increased reactivity and a narrowing of the breathing passages. This reaction is transient and when the attack is over, the airway passages return to normal, allowing air to enter and exit the lungs normally.

The incidence of asthma decreases with age. The exact cause of asthma is not known, but external factors can influence and worsen the symptoms, including cold air, dry air, dust, exercise, air pollution, medications (aspirin, antibiotics) and allergens (pollen, pets). Episodes of asthma may vary in intensity from person to person, ranging from mild "tightness" or wheezing of the chest to extremely severely restricted airways providing very little air movement into the lungs—a life-threatening condition requiring immediate medical attention. These episodes can also vary in duration lasting from minutes to hours of restricted breathing.

Asthma is a very common medical condition shared by many children. According to a 2004 report from the American Lung Association, four million children under eighteen had an asthma attack in a twelve-month time period; many others may have had "hidden" or undiagnosed asthma.

Children who need surgery and have asthma will ideally need to have excellent medical control of it prior to a procedure as they may be prone to attacks before, during and after surgery. Stress alone, though rare, can play a large part. Relief is sometimes quick and simple, with the right medications, though sometimes, an attack can take hours to bring under control. The better the asthma is controlled before surgery, the less likely it is for the patient to experience an asthma attack under anesthesia.

- **If your child has asthma, it is very important that you carry all asthma medications with you, specifically all inhalers, when you take your child to the hospital for surgery.** If an asthma attack occurs during surgery, the anesthesiologist will use intravenous, inhalational and/or subcutaneous (injection under the skin with a very thin needle) routes to manage the exacerbation of the asthma. The anesthesiologist has all necessary means to best treat and stop an asthma attack if one should occur during surgery.

- **If your child has asthma, it is also important that you ensure that he or she take all preventative medications, as recommended by his or her physician, prior to going to the hospital for surgery.** This may include the rescue medications atrovent or albuterol, or any other inhaler that may be recommended by your child's physician.

On occasion, an asthmatic may develop symptoms immediately after surgery due to the cold, dry gases used during surgery. An anesthesiologist can take certain preventative measures, such as the use of rehumidification filters, to keep the air your child breathes during surgery as warm and moist as possible, to reduce further triggering of an asthma attack. In the recovery room, humidified oxygen may also be administered, to help treat or reduce the likelihood of an asthma attack.

Head Colds and Runny Noses

Head colds or other upper respiratory tract infections could raise the risk of a reaction to anesthetic, particularly if there is a related fever or cough with mucous secretions. These conditions may increase the sensitivity of the airway passage lining and increase the likelihood of a reaction similar to the one seen in patients with asthma. A progressive narrowing or spasm of the airway passages can occur as a result of the interaction of cold medical gases with the lining of the lungs. This would make the passage of oxygen difficult.

Your child's physician and anesthesiologist will evaluate your child thoroughly if there is any suspicion that there may be an increased risk with the anesthetic. The safety of the child comes first and if this is an elective procedure that can be performed at a later date under safer conditions, the physicians may make the decision to postpone the procedure until a time when it could be done under safer circumstances.

An exception to this option may include:

- An infection related to the medical condition that is to be corrected surgically.

- An urgent procedure that cannot wait for the resolution of the infection.

In either case, the surgeon and the anesthesiologist will evaluate the child and determine the optimum circumstances, to ensure the safest and best outcome.

Some children almost always have runny noses without really being "sick." In the absence of fever or lethargy, surgery and anesthesia have been shown to be safe in these children.

Diabetes

Diabetes mellitus is a sugar metabolism disorder distinguished by the inability to incorporate glucose, the body's main energy source, into the cells of the body. There are two types of diabetes:

- Type I (juvenile diabetes)—13,000 children are diagnosed with type I diabetes each year. This disorder involves the destruction of a type of cell in the pancreas that is responsible for the secretion of insulin, which helps in the metabolism of glucose. Initial symptoms may include extreme thirst and increased frequency of urination. The high level of sugar in the blood gets dumped into the urine through the kidneys, thus draining large quantities of fluid from within the body. The poorly controlled glucose in the blood causes greater fluid loss and gives rise to dehydration and thirst. Type I diabetes is usually treated through self- or assisted injection of insulin. Blood sugar measurements are also usually self-monitored by a finger stick and the use of standardized chemical strips obtained from a pharmacy.

- Type II (adult onset)—now accounts for eight percent of childhood diabetics. This disorder is characterized by increasing issues with poor weight control and by the body's resistance to the effects of insulin. Treatment can include dietary restriction, oral medication and/or insulin.

Blood glucose monitoring and insulin administration is a life-long process to ensure proper blood sugar control. Poor blood sugar control accelerates the risk of heart disease, kidney failure, loss of vision and nerve injury in the extremities, among other issues.

Blood sugar control is particularly important during the time surrounding surgery, because high sugar can interfere with healing and increase the risk of infection.

- Please have your child visit a pediatrician and an endocrinologist regularly prior to the surgery, in the event that the insulin dose needs to be adjusted to ensure tighter blood sugar control and monitoring.

- Follow the physician's recommendations closely. If your child has diabetes, he or she may need to be admitted to the hospital in advance of the surgery for close monitoring of the glucose.

Glucose levels in the blood can be impacted by dietary restrictions, anxiety and the stress of surgery, and require close monitoring. During the surgery itself, the anesthesiologist will monitor the glucose levels. The release of adrenaline associated with the stress of surgery could make the blood sugar levels swing widely, depending on the circumstances.

Remember, **the tighter the blood sugar control prior to the start of the surgery, the less risk of severe changes in blood sugar during the procedure.** Please follow your physician's recommendations closely.

Obesity

Obesity is becoming an increasing concern among the young population, partially due to a shift in diet and lifestyle. Our culture's recent emphasis on changing our diets to fit into fast, ready-made meals has compromised the nutritional value of what we eat.

Fast food chains have fed into this frenzy by maximizing portions and indirectly encouraging parents and children alike to consume monster-sized burgers and fries, with giant portions of sugar-rich soda. This fad has also been complicated by the advent of the technological age—children are spending less time exercising in free play such as tag and pick-up sports. They now spend more time in sedentary endeavors such as instant messaging, cell phone conversations or computer use.

Obesity is giving rise to an entire series of medical conditions that will plague our children for the rest of their lives. Weight related medical conditions include diabetes, heart disease, breathing problems, circulatory problems, gastrointestinal issues and neurological issues.

Obese individuals:

• Develop resistance to the action of insulin, which throws

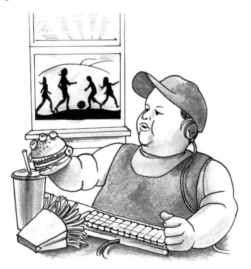

off the normal blood sugar metabolism. The body breaks down most starch into glucose, which is a simple sugar used by the body for energy. Insulin helps move glucose into cells, where it can be utilized to create energy for the cell. Obesity predisposes many children to type II diabetes. Since they become resistant to insulin, other treatments need to be applied in order to obtain better blood sugar control, such as proper diet and physical exercise, which are important when attempting to reverse the abnormal metabolic process. Weight control is a lifelong disciplinary process that along with diet, needs to be conducted under the directions of a physician and nutritionist.

- Have an increased requirement of oxygen metabolism and production of carbon dioxide from their increased mass. This process taxes the circulatory system, including the heart and lungs; the heart works harder while trying to circulate more oxygen-rich blood throughout the body, while the lungs work to get rid of the toxic carbon dioxide created by the breakdown of glucose. The lungs also bring more oxygen to the blood from the air. But this becomes difficult with increased weight around the chest and abdomen, which can press against the lungs and interfere with their full expansion, making them extremely inefficient. The heart can experience resistance in the flow of the blood through the restricted volume of the lungs, and through larger-than-usual body mass when moving the blood around the circulatory system. This can cause high blood pressure, which can contribute to further compromising of the heart and other organs.

- Can develop sleep apnea. Some of the mass surrounding the face and neck can interfere with normal movement of air into the lungs. This becomes significant when an obese person sleeps, as it can compromise oxygen delivery to the organs. After a sleep study, if sleep apnea is suspected, special steps may need to be taken to ensure that there is no compromise of air flow while the patient is being induced to sleep with anesthesia, or awakening from anesthesia. Special devices—such as continuous positive airway pressure (CPAP) machines, which are designed to keep airway passages open through the application of pressure through a small mask that fits over the nose or mouth—can help maintain continuous air flow as a person recovering from anesthesia or sleeping at home. It is very likely that children suspected of having of having sleep apnea will need to spend the night in the hospital following a procedure, for observational and safety purposes.

- Have increased stomach acid levels and larger stomach volume. With increasing weight, there is progressive pressure within the abdomen and abnormal slowing of intestinal functioning. This interferes with the rate at which the stomach empties into the intestine, increasing the volume of the stomach's contents. These factors increase the risk of a condition known as aspiration pneumonitis (inhalation of stomach contents into the lungs) during surgery. It is important to follow all dietary restriction guidelines prior to surgery to decrease the risk of this condition.

All of the above factors play an important role in contributing to the risks of surgery for any child. While it is true that some of these factors can be modified or helped, others are part of a life-long process of controlling the effects of obesity.

Additional Risks

The body has a natural tendency to decrease efforts to breathe following surgery; this occurs because of splinting, as a result of pain and other factors. This can further increase the risk of collapse of the small air sacks in the lungs, giving rise to the development of pneumonia. Good pain control regimens following surgery, with motivated deep-breathing exercises directed by the nursing care staff, will help reduce this risk. Mobility and movement, under the direction of the physician, will also help reduce the risk of blood clot formation in the lower extremities.

It is important to follow a physician's directions for weight control, whether they come from your child's pediatrician or surgeon. Following their recommendations and encouraging good nutrition in your child can help reduce the likelihood of potential issues that may create a risk during your child's surgery.

Chapter 13
Allergies and Drug Sensitivity

What You Need to Be Aware Of

Understanding Allergies

An allergy is defined as any immunologic (involving the immune system) response to a particular substance. An allergic reaction indicates that the body, for some reason or another, has developed antibodies toward a medication or other allergen (a substance that causes an allergic reaction) that the body has been exposed to previously. Once the body is exposed to the allergen again, the immune system is triggered.

Most drug allergies are rare, but penicillin is the most common medication a person may become allergic to. Today, the incidence of this allergy is estimated to be less than ten percent.

It is important that you, as a parent, document any and all reactions your child may develop to any suspected medications.

If your child does have and adverse reaction to a medication, take notes and keep them with your child's medical records. Within your notes about the incident, include:

- The name of the medication

- The type of reaction (rash, itch, hives, fever)

- The extent of the reaction (small area, which part of the body, the entire body)

- The time between exposure to the medication and the reaction

- The duration of the reaction

- The type and effectiveness of the treatment

Note: It is not sufficient to rely on your pediatrician to maintain this information accurately. This information may not be readily available when necessary—particularly years down the road, when the child has grown, or at a time of emergency. Keep this information at your fingertips; it could save your child's life and provide to be invaluable information for his or her care in the future.

It is vital that you inform your child's surgeon and anesthesiologist of any and all past allergic reactions to medications, as well as environmental and food allergies, including shellfish.

If your child has an allergy to shellfish, there is a possibility that there can be a reaction to a type of contrast chemical used to enhance images in special diagnostic X-rays. Please clarify this with your physician before consenting to any X-rays that could involve injection of contrast media or contrast dye.

Allergic reactions to medications (or anything else) can be mild to severe, ranging from itch, rash, redness, hives, flushing or swelling anywhere on the body. Swelling of the throat can make breathing difficult due to the release of certain chemicals in the body including histamine, leukotrienes and prostoglandins. Some of these chemical reactions occur with hay fever and other environmental allergies. These chemicals can act locally or enter the blood stream and act systemically (throughout the body). Aside from swelling, these chemicals can contribute to a significant decrease in blood pressure, which can reduce the flow of blood to vital organs.

In rare instances, when an allergic reaction leads to swelling around the throat that interferes with breathing, a medical condition known as anaphylactic shock can arise. It is important to present any detailed information regarding medication reactions to your physician prior to care to help avoid such severe, dangerous circumstances for your child.

Reactions to Medications

Allergic reactions to medications do not generally occur on the first exposure to the medication. Usually, allergy occurs on a subsequent dosing of the same medication. The body, for some reason, recognizes the medication as a foreign body and develops antibodies on a first exposure; on the following exposure, these antibodies are released to fight off the offending agent, thus triggering an allergic reaction.

If there have been any prior reactions to any medications, it is important that you let your physician differentiate between a true allergic reaction and a common side effect (intolerance) of the medication, such as nausea and vomiting. Improper classification of a reaction can interfere with the use of similar medications that may be useful in the care of your child. Don't attempt to make this assumption on your own; your child's physician will discuss this with you and make the decision regarding a specific medication.

Allergy or Intolerance?

Many times, the symptoms of allergies and side effects (intolerance) are confused. For instance, those who take erythromycin as an antibiotic and experience loose bowel movements or nausea are not allergic to erythromycin, but experience an unpleasant side effect of the medication. The same applies to other medications. Side effects such as nausea and vomiting may be confused with and often described as allergies. Ask your pediatrician to help you differentiate between an allergic reaction and a side effect of a medication.

Chapter 14
Blood Transfusions

What Is the Potential for Blood Loss Necessitating Blood Transfusion?

One of the most common concerns surrounding surgery is the potential for blood loss that may necessitate a transfusion. But, keep in mind that it is extremely rare for a healthy child to need a blood transfusion for any of the common surgical procedures performed today, and every effort is made by the healthcare professionals involved in the surgery to reduce the risks of the need for a blood transfusion.

When Is a Blood Transfusion Needed?

The need for a blood transfusion may increase in patients requiring extensive surgery, particularly if it involves large blood vessels or organs that receive large amount of blood flow—situations that may create a greater risk of blood loss. The need for a blood transfusion will also depend on the health of the child and whether or not he or she is able to tolerate blood loss.

Can My Child Give His or Her Own Blood Before Surgery?

With today's improved technology, we are able to use cell savers, complex machines comprised of independent suction devices used in combination with centrifuges and filtration systems. In certain instances and with certain types of procedures, blood can be removed through suction tubing. The red blood cells can then be separated out of the blood, washed, concentrated and then returned to a transfusion bag, which can be used to return the blood to the patient during or shortly after the procedure. However, there are instances wherein the cell saver device has limitations and cannot be used.

Depending on the health and age of your child, the physician may be able to perform autologous blood transfusions. If the surgery is planned in advance, an older child may be able to donate small amounts of his or her own blood that can be stored in the blood bank for a very short period of time, in preparation for the surgery. Again, this can vary depending on the type of surgery and the health and age of your child, among other circumstances.

The risks and benefits of blood transfusion and blood product therapy (discussed later in this chapter) are weighed very carefully prior to any determination for such a procedure. If the surgical procedure or the personal health status of the child poses the potential for significant blood loss, an effort will be made to provide medical care that will not only conserve the child's blood, but provide a means by which transfusion will be safe, should the need arise.

To help you to understand why someone might need a blood transfusion, let me first discuss the function of the blood in the body, and the risks involved if the blood supply is depleted to unacceptable levels.

The Function of Blood in the Body

What are RBCs?

Red blood cells (RBCs) carry oxygen to all parts of the body. This maintains the metabolism of the body and energy production in combination with glucose (sugar). The body requires a minimum of a certain concentration of RBCs, also known as the hematocrit or hemoglobin level, to do this safely.

The hematocrit level is determined after a blood sample is taken. The vial of blood is spun in a device known as a centrifuge. The RBCs settle to the bottom of the vial because they are heavier than the fluid that surrounds them. The hematocrit is a percentage of the RBCs to the total fluid volume in the vial.

The lowest necessary percentage of hematocrit in the blood varies from person to person and is affected by many underlying medical conditions. Most clinicians view twenty-five percent as the lower end of the limit, but this number is not absolute and again depends on the unique set of circumstances at hand.

The RBC level is determined by a simple pre-operative

blood test known as the complete blood count (CBC). That number helps determine how much blood loss a child may be able to withstand without risking serous complications, including death. It is the main role of the physicians involved in the surgical care of the child to determine this factor.

What Else Is Blood Made Of?

Human blood also contains important components necessary for clotting. These components help seal cut veins, preventing further blood loss.

The components include:

- Platelets: small cells, derived from bone marrow, that cling together, helping in the clotting process.

- Proteins that help construct a fine mesh along the edges of cut blood vessels, where platelets can cling and further help clot formation.

Blood tests that are part of normal pre-operative testing can determine if your child's clotting abilities are within a normal. Most healthy children may not require the entire range of tests and may only need the test to determine the concentration of RBCs. If there is any medical history of easy bruising, bleeding from the gums when brushing teeth, or prolonged nose bleeds, your child may require additional blood tests in addition to the basic CBC.

What Is the CBC Blood Test?

The Complete blood count (CBC) is a test that will show

actual levels of the RBCs, WBCs, platelets, hemoglobin and hematocrit. White blood cells (WBC) are the body's defense—they fight off infection. Hemoglobin (Hb) is the iron-containing oxygen transport protein contained in the RBC. Hematocrit (Ht or HCT) is the proportion of RBCs to the total blood volume.

In conjunction with a CBC, two other tests, prothrombin time (PT) and partial thromboplastin time (PTT) are also run. These tests look at two different clotting mechanisms that involve proteins outside of platelets that take part in the clotting of blood.

Additional testing and treatment may be necessary if there are concerns about blood clotting in genetically inherited diseases, such as certain types of hemophilia. These genetic conditions result in clotting issues due to defects in the generation of certain proteins necessary for clotting factors.

Any of the blood to be used for transfusion is screened using chemical analysis known as ELISA and Western blot techniques, which are the standard and most current techniques for finding HIV as well as hepatitis B and C viral infections. Multiple scientific studies have shown the rate of transmission of HIV to be 1 in 128,000; HBV (hepatitis B) is shown to be 1 in 63,000 and HCV (hepatitis C) is shown to be 1 in 103,000. These numbers are for all blood transfusions.

Blood transfusion is a necessary component of any surgery, if substantial blood loss occurs. But, compared to the list of other potential risks, including including death and irreversible organ damage from serious levels of blood loss (as discussed earlier), the risk of transmission of infection during a blood transfusion is considered very low. To further reduce the risk of blood reactions and transmission of infectious agents, the pharmaceutical industry is conducting studies to develop a synthetic substitute.

Any blood that is donated is screened to keep detectable

life-threatening viruses from contaminating the blood supply. Keep in mind that blood is a vulnerable and rare commodity today. Specific criteria are followed with regard to transfusion and proper allocation of blood for those who really need this life-saving therapy. If your child receives a transfusion, you can be sure that his or her health and/or life are viewed to be at serious risk.

How Does the Hospital Know My Child's Blood Type?

Blood cells carry antigens—protein molecules that identify the cells as unique to that individual and can potentially cause a severe reaction in another person. There are four recognized blood type groups: A, B, AB and O. The presence of a specific protein called Rhesus (Rh) antigen makes a person positive and the absence makes a person negative. Thus, a blood type has two components: a letter (A, B, AB, O) and an Rh component (positive or negative).

A blood bank identifies donor and recipient blood types by identifying the antigens in the blood, and potential reactions by "cross matching" the blood of the donor with that of the recipient. It is a trial blood transfusion in a test tube, to see if there are any adverse reactions. This is done in three phases:

1. Introduction or intermediate phase—an evaluation of any reaction that may occur within one to five minutes and determines errors in ABO typing.

2. Incubation phase—the incubation of the mixture at body temperature for ten to thirty minutes, depending

on the types of solutions used for the reaction. This phase is designed to help detect any reactions that may be outside of the ABO groups.

3. Antiglobulin phase—the adding of an antiglobulin (protein) sera to the mixture to detect any additional incompatibilities.

With these arduous tests, it is very rare for an allergic or other type of reaction to occur as a result of a transfusion. I have described the process of blood typing to impress upon you that it is not an instantaneous process; it requires some time for the entire process to take place. Before any determination for a transfusion takes place, a blood sample will be taken from your child, to determine his or her blood type and to help reduce any possible risk of a blood reaction.

Blood Products Therapy

Blood is a very valuable resource and is often in short supply. With the use of modern technology, blood has been broken down into its various components so that individuals whose blood may lack specific components can be specifically treated, and the unneeded components can be saved for others who could use them.

Blood is usually broken down to three major components: PRBCs, platelets and fresh frozen plasma (FFP).

PRBCs (packed red blood cells) are a composite of red blood cells in a solution designed to keep them viable for greater than thirty days. They are used in a person with excessive bleeding who needs red blood cells to maintain adequate oxygen delivery to his or her vital organs.

Platelets are given to a person who has a deficiency of platelets as a result of a disease process, or as a result of large-volume transfusions (for example, someone who is involved in a traumatic injury). Large-volume transfusions could decrease the effectiveness of clotting.

FFP (fresh frozen plasma) is the portion of the blood that is void of any red blood cells and platelets. It may resemble straw-colored lemonade. It is used in people who have clotting disorders as a result of any of a variety of medical conditions, or due to medications.

Whole blood is used in someone who needs blood because of blood loss and suffers from a clotting dysfunction as well. Your child's surgeon will discuss in detail with you if your child should be at any risk for needing a blood transfusion.

I know that it's a very stressful time in your life. I hope that some of these recommendations prove to be helpful as you embark on the surgical journey with your child. It is my intention to help make this journey as smooth as possible.

Section IV
COMMONLY PERFORMED PEDIATRIC SURGERIES

Chapter 15
General Guidelines

What Can You Expect During a Surgical Day?

Some General Guidelines

Within this chapter, I will review some common pediatric surgical procedures and present general guidelines for each of the surgeries, to give you an idea of what to expect if your child should have any of these problems.

This guide is not intended to help you diagnose your child, or to assist you in treating your child's medical condition. The procedures that I discuss below have been extremely simplified to help you understand the underlying mechanics of how a surgical day may unfold and in general, what you can expect to take place during a specific type of surgery. The actual mechanism of how each medical condition is diagnosed and treated, how surgery is performed, how each child is anesthetized and awakened, and how the child recovers after surgery, involves many complex steps. Each step is orchestrated with professional service to ensure the best possible outcome.

A small guide of this type will not be able to describe or replace any one of those steps, let alone shortcut the many years of education and training your physician has gone through. Each child is different, and each medical condition needs to be evaluated by a trained physician on an individual basis, so that the decisions made are in the best interests of the child and will help ensure a good outcome. Be assured that most healthcare providers strive for perfection and that nothing less than a perfect outcome for your child will be acceptable to them.

SPECIFIC PEDIATRIC SURGICAL PROCEDURES

Adenoidectomy

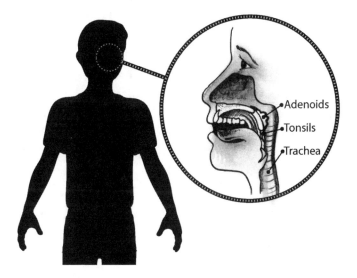

Causes

The adenoids are spongy tissue that is part of the immune system. Located in the upper rear of the throat, where the nasal passages are, the adnoids are similiar in appearance and function to the tonsils.

They help fight certain infections in children up to the age of three to five years, and can swell as a result of infection, depending on the fequency and type.

Swollen adenoids can cause certain problems in the child, from interfering with the ease of breathing to frequent ear infections. Often, the adenoids can cause problems in conjunction with the tonsils, which are a similar tissue located in the back of the throat. It is rare that only the adenoids will be removed without removing the tonsils. Approximately 250,000 combination tonsillectomy/adenoidectomy procedures are performed each year, compared to only about 15,000 adenoidectomy-only procedures.

The Procedure

If there is an infection associated with the adenoids, every attempt will be made to minimize the level of the infection prior to surgery, by treating the child with antibiotics.

Prior to surgery, the child's diet will be restricted as described earlier in this book except for some types of clear liquids, depending on the anesthesiologist's preference. The surgeon and the anesthesiologist will meet with you and your child prior to the procedure and discuss the plan and what to expect.

Depending on the medical center where your child will be having surgery, you may be allowed to dress in the required garb and follow your child into the operating room, to assist him or her with drifting off to sleep. While your child is asleep, the surgeon will use various instruments to remove the enlarged adenoid tissue and control the bleeding. Once the surgeon can determine the effectiveness of the removal of the adenoids, he will ensure that there is adequate control of the bleeding and will indicate that the surgery is over. At that point, the anesthesiologist will begin to bring the child out of the anesthesia.

Anesthesia

After you enter the operating room with your child, depending on his or her age, a clear plastic mask filled with oxygen and anesthetic gases may be applied over your child's nose and mouth, to help him or her drift off to a gentle sleep. If the child is older, medication will be injected through an IV.

On occasion, a child will struggle a bit while breathing in anesthetic gases from the mask. This is normal as the child's conscious state drifts and enters the various stages of anesthesia. Once the child is asleep, you will be asked to leave the operating room and the procedure will be performed.

A breathing tube is used for this procedure, to protect the windpipe. The surgeon may elect to inject the area with local anesthetic to either help reduce the amount of bleeding during the surgery or help with pain relief following surgery. There are various schools of thought on the injection of local anesthetic, because as it wears off, so do the effects of the adrenaline, and this has the potential to increase the risk of bleeding during the child's recovery. Depending on the circumstances, the surgeon will determine the best course of action.

After the procedure is completed, the anesthesiologist will remove the breathing tube as the child emerges from anesthesia. It is important that the child's ability to protect his or her windpipe by coughing and swallowing return when this breathing apparatus is removed, to help the lungs function effectively. Sufficient anesthetic will remain within the circulatory system, and this will cause the child to have no or very little memory of the awakening process.

PACU

Most children cry upon emergence from anesthesia, which helps with sufficient breathing. When this happens, we do not rush to treat the child with pain medications because the crying is not necessarily due to pain; it could also be due to anxiety, fear, an emotionally liable state associated with surgery, anesthesia, waking up in an unfamiliar setting and so forth.

Pain medications can also disguise or mask potentially dangerous settings associated with bleeding, and circumstances that can interfere with breathing.

Before pain medication is dispensed to a screaming child, a great deal of thought and consideration goes into the evaluation. The surgeon and the PACU staff may elect to observe the child for a few hours because of concerns with bleeding or breathing issues. These steps are precautions to provide maximum safety for the child before discharge.

Risks

There are four primary risks associated with an adenoidectomy:

- Breathing—because of the location of the surgery, in or near the back of the throat. Once the breathing tube has been situated, there is a very minor risk of breathing issues. The anesthesiologist monitors this closely, to ensure that there are adequate breaths delivered. He or she uses a variety of monitors that show the volume of the breaths delivered, the concentration of the oxygen, the pressure of the breaths delivered and the amount of carbon dioxide that is exhaled. This information is readily available with each breath, to ensure that the appropriate intervention is employed immediately, should it be necessary. Be assured that your child is very safe with this type of technology at hand. Breathing may be a concern in the PACU, observing the child to ensure that the anesthetic wears off adequately and swelling does not interfere with breathing.

• Bleeding—the mouth and throat contain large number of blood vessels. Bleeding is not only a concern during surgery, but also immediately after surgery. The PACU staff is trained to watch for increased risks of bleeding, and your patience is greatly appreciated while you wait until your child is adequately recovered prior to being discharged.

• Nausea—a mild risk in patients who had surgery in the nose, throat or ear areas. Traces of blood may be swallowed after surgery, which can cause nausea. The PACU staff will evaluate each child for nausea and ensure that it is well-controlled prior to discharge.

• Infection—you may need to monitor your child's temperature following surgery for signs of infection. When your child is discharged, monitor him or her closely and follow the instructions the PACU staff will provide.

Contact your child's surgeon immediately if you notice any of the following:

• Changes in the pattern of breathing—a rapid and shallow manner.

• Drastic behavioral change—your child becomes more languid.

• Increased bleeding in the back of the throat—if your child spits up bright-red blood.

• The development of a fever.

If any of these occur, please contact your surgeon immediately and prepare your child to return to the hospital immediately, because these may be signs of impaired breathing due to bleeding or swelling.

The PACU staff may provide you with instructions for your child upon discharge. He or she may be restricted to either liquids or a very soft diet in the first forty-eight to seventy-two hours. Each physician may have his or her own concerns and guidelines regarding the advancement of diet. Please follow their instructions closely to ensure the best and safest outcome for your child, and to minimize the risk of bleeding and infection.

Appendectomy

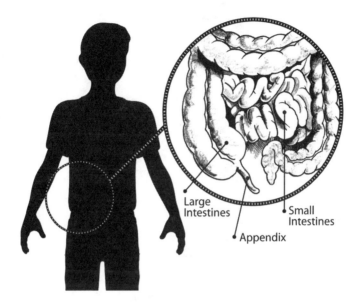

Large
Intestines

Small
Intestines

Appendix

Causes

The appendix plays no role in the human body—it is a non-functioning, very small portion of intestine that remains as part of our digestive system, located at the juncture of the small and large intestines. The size of the appendix varies in diameter and length but is usually approximately the size of a pinky finger. Usually, it is located in the right lower abdomen, halfway to two-thirds of the way between the bellybutton and right groin. This location can change depending on anatomic variations.

For unknown reasons, the appendix often becomes inflamed, causing various symptoms from vague abdominal pain to nausea, fever and fatigue. Appendicitis is extremely rare in infants, but if it happens, their symptoms may include vomiting, diarrhea and possibly a swollen abdomen.

Children under the age five may only complain of abdominal pain or hold their bellies. The pain may begin near the belly button and migrate toward the right side of the abdomen. Children with this problem usually lack any appetite or desire to eat. The symptoms can also be vague and mimic other medical conditions. A child who exhibits these symptoms needs to seek prompt medical attention, as the danger of a ruptured appendicitis is significant.

There has been a slow change in the protocol of treating appendicitis with high doses of antibiotics, depending on regional and hospital protocols. The landscape of treatment protocols for all types of diseases tends to change with advancement of knowledge, new technology and ongoing pressure from health insurance companies. Your child's physician will review with you the best course of treatment for your child.

The appendix has a thin wall, and an inflamed appendix is teeming with bacteria. A ruptured appendix can spread infection rapidly throughout the abdomen, with consequences that are wide and potentially dangerous—even deadly.

A child with appendicitis symptoms is often evaluated in the emergency department by the on-call surgeon. If appendicitis is suspected, preparations will be made for surgery.

Things may move quickly if surgery is planned:

- The surgeon will contact the operating room and arrange for a time for the procedure, which can be considered an emergency depending on how much the infection has progressed. Most hospitals reserve one room for such emergencies; other hospitals will piggyback the procedure to whatever operating room finishes its scheduled operations first.

- The operating room will be prepared. If other procedures of less urgency were previously scheduled, they will be postponed or moved to other less-busy operating rooms, later in the day. Often, an individual with appendicitis will initially be treated with antibiotics and followed closely to see if there is improvement of symptoms. These determinations will be made by your child's physician.

> It is not wise to force a child to eat; forced eating can contribute to a variety of issues and complications surrounding the time of surgery.
> See page 43
> PLEASE follow the instructions provided by the medical professionals closely.

The Procedure

Parents are seldom allowed to enter the operating room for emergency procedures. There are many professional personnel standing by to manage the urgency of the procedure and aside from the pediatric anesthesiologist, there may be additional anesthesia providers standing by to assist as the child is drifting off to sleep. Depending on the age, an IV may be placed, usually in the arm, if this was not already done in the emergency department to replenish fluids that the child may have lost from lack of oral intake and loss of fluids from fever, diarrhea and vomiting.

Once the child is asleep, the surgeon will clean the area of the abdomen with antibacterial soap and place sterile drapes around it. The surgery may be performed in one of two ways:

- Traditionally—making the incision in the area above the appendix.

- Via laparoscopy—using small incisions in the abdomen to introduce two or three thin, telescoping instruments into the abdomen. One of these instruments contains a light and a camera, which help the surgeon visualize the inside of the abdomen on a television monitor. The surgeon makes an incision and controls the bleeding as he descends through the various layers of skin, fat and muscle, to enter the abdominal cavity. Once he or she reaches the abdominal cavity, the condition of the appendix and surrounding tissues are evaluated to see the extent of the infection. If the appendix is intact, it is carefully isolated from the surrounding tissues to minimize the risk of rupture while the procedure proceeds. If the procedure is performed in the traditional open technique, the appendix will appear swollen, red and stiff, and feel warm to the touch. (There is no direct contact with the appendix when surgery is performed by laparoscopy). The appendix is usually then clamped or sutured at the base and removed from the abdominal cavity. If the appendix is ruptured, then an attempt is made to isolate the infection, and the infected appendix is removed. The abdominal cavity is usually cleansed with antibiotic solution to wash away bacterial contamination and minimize the risk of spreading the infection. Once the appendix is removed, and the abdomen is evaluated and deemed free of infection by the surgeon, the abdomen is closed, the dressing is applied and the patient is allowed to emerge from the anesthetic.

Anesthesia

Most of the time, parents will not be allowed into the operating room because the sequence of events will differ in comparison to an elective procedure, and there may be no time to properly dress a parent and orient them to the circumstances.

When there is a question as to whether the medical condition has impacted the normal function of the intestines and stomach, another anesthesia provider will participate in a technique referred to as a rapid sequence induction (RSI) with cricoid pressure. This method of anesthesia induction is reserved for surgical procedures that are emergent in nature, or have less- than-ideal circumstances wherein the stomach is not completely empty. A clear plastic mask is placed over the child's face and nose and filled with one-hundred-percent oxygen. Ordinary room air oxygen only contains twenty-one percent oxygen, which in comparison, is like driving around with less than a quarter tank of gasoline. Once the injected medications cause the breathing to stop, there needs to be as much oxygen in the lungs as possible until the anesthesiologist can secure and control the breathing.

Simultaneously, the second anesthesia provider will exert gentle pressure against the windpipe, over cricoid cartilage. The windpipe has cartilaginous rings in it; the cricoid cartilage is the first ring that completely surrounds the windpipe. By pressing against it, a seal is formed against the esophagus, reducing the likelihood of any acid or stomach contents regurgitating up into the opening of the windpipe or the larynx.

If the procedure is not deemed urgent, then you may be allowed into the operating room. It is always up to the anesthesiologist's discretion, depending on the urgency of the situation. General anesthesia is the anesthetic used for this procedure and oxygen will be given through a clear plastic mask as intravenous agents are infused into the arm, to help the child drift off to sleep. A breathing tube will be placed to ultimately protect the windpipe and through which to administer breaths.

Near the conclusion of the procedure, the surgeon may inject local anesthesia into the wound to help prolong pain relief following the procedure.

PACU

After the child emerges from anesthesia and the breathing tube is removed, he or she will be taken to the PACU. The child will probably be groggy as he or she continues to wake up but will be evaluated by the nursing staff as recovery progresses. The staff will administer pain medications and other medications if needed, for example, should the child become nauseated. The child will recover in the hospital, receiving a full compliment of intravenous antibiotics after the removal of the infected appendix.

The post-surgery diet usually begins with clear liquids once there are indications that the intestines have resumed normal activity. The intestines usually slow or stop in function when the abdomen is disturbed due to surgery, and may need up to twenty-four to forty-eight hours to resume activity. Clear liquids are the first form of nutrition; the diet will be advanced as the child begins to tolerate more and more.

Risks

The major issue revolving around an appendectomy is the risk of a ruptured appendix, as I discussed above.

Aside from infection, bleeding is always a concern when surgery is performed. Despite the urgency, all precautions are taken during surgery to ensure proper control of any bleeding.

Certain conditions may contribute to the increased risk of bleeding:

- If the infection has spread and caused an interference with the clotting factors, due to severe shock brought on by a delay in seeking medical care

• If the child has certain conditions that affect the clotting factors and may prolong bleeding, such as hemophilia or idiopathic thrombocy-topenic purpura.

The intestines slow or stop in function during an appendicitis attack, and this contributes to the lack of appetite and nausea. The stomach is considered full, and there is a risk of reflux or regurgitation during the anesthesia. There is always a hazard of the stomach contents entering the windpipe under these circumstances. It is important not to encourage any intake of food if the child is experiencing abdominal discomfort or nausea of this type.

Cleft Lip and Palate Repair

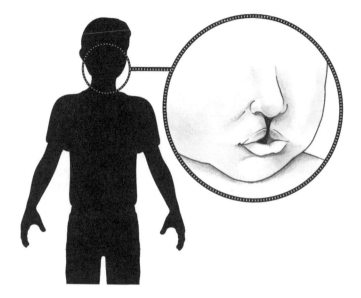

Causes

Cleft palate is caused by incomplete or nondevelopment of the various parts of the plates that merge to form the roof of the mouth, lips, throat or various parts of the nasal and oral passages. This defect can involve the skin, the lining of the mucosa or delicate, moist lining inside the mouth and nose, or the bony plates of the hard palate, in varying degrees.

Cleft palate can not only be visibly disfiguring, but it can contribute to various issues with swallowing, speech, breathing and recurring infections involving the ears and sinuses. The surgery to correct this defect is designed to: 1) help return function so that the child is able to eat, drink, develop speech and breathe without any hindrance and 2) help correct the disfiguring aspect.

Depending on the degree of the defect, the surgery will be performed at different stages of the child's development because the plan for surgery will take into consideration the growth of the child's face. This type of surgical procedure is usually performed by an ear nose and throat (ENT) surgeon or by a plastic surgeon who specializes in the correction of facial deformities. The surgeon will evaluate the degree of defect and determine the proper approach, and decide if the surgery will require revisions or corrections as the child grows. Orthodontics may play a role at some point as well, to help the teeth grow as normally as possible.

The Procedure

Once the child has drifted off to sleep, the surgeon will clean the affected area with antiseptic soap and begin the procedure. If the defect only involves a small area of the lip, nasal fold or soft palate, then the repair may only require an incision and closure of the defect. If the problem is more extensive, the surgery may involve various steps to correct underlying defects, which can include taking grafts or tissue flaps from neighboring or other parts of the body to rebuild the architecture of the base of the nasal floor or roof of the mouth, or to correct large defects involving the lips and other oral structures. The surgery is delicate and may involve many hours of reconstructive surgery.

Usually, the child will be awakened in the operating room and transported to the PACU. If the surgery is extensive and requires many hours to complete, or if it involves a correction of larger defects or vast correction near the back of the throat, then the child might need to be transferred to the intensive care unit (ICU) after surgery for close observation.

Anesthesia

Parents will usually be permitted to proceed with their child to the operating room. General anesthesia is preferred for these procedures. Depending on the age of the child, a clear mask filled with anesthetic gases may be applied to the face, to help him or her drift off to sleep. If an IV is available or if the child allows the placement of the IV, it will be utilized to help the child drift off to sleep.

After the parent has been escorted from the room, a breathing tube will be placed into the child's windpipe, to protect the lungs and to ensure oxygen delivery and breathing during surgery. In most cases, the breathing tube will be removed as the child awakens. In cases wherein the swelling of the surgical area may interfere with breathing, the breathing tube will be left in place, to ensure breathing. The child will be transferred to the ICU for close observation until the swelling resolves and the breathing tube is removed.

PACU

Once in the PACU or ICU, nurses will observe the child closely for potential bleeding and for swelling that may impede breathing. The majority of patients who undergo this surgery stay in the hospital for a few days not only for observation, but because there is a significant risk of infection and bleeding following surgery.

The mouth can harbor a variety of bacteria with the potential to cause an infection, and the child may need to be on antibiotics to reduce this risk. The mouth is extremely vascular, meaning that the structure receives a large volume of blood flow. If there is any risk of the disruption of the blood vessels in the fresh surgical wound, bleeding can contribute to swelling.

Diet is crucial to the child recovering from cleft palate surgery. When fully awake, the child will be started on liquids and then slowly progress to a soft diet. The texture of certain types of foods can increase the risk of bleeding or swelling.

Risks

We touched upon some of the risks associated with cleft palate repair above, including bleeding due to the vascular nature of the oral and nasal cavities, and infection due to all the different types of bacteria that inhabit the mouth.

The surgical procedure involving the repair of a cleft palate, tongue, lips or nose is complex, depending on the severity of the defect. In this procedure, the surgeon brings together the separated flaps of tissue. If they are connected to tightly, there can be complications, the connection can come undone, the underlying blood flow can be compromised, or the blood vessels can burst from being under too much stress. Because of this degree of difficulty, a great deal of planning goes into the procedure. Post-surgery, the wound will require close observation by the healthcare staff. Your child will most likely be cared for in an intensive care unit until swelling from the procedure subsides and his or her situation improves.

The patient will also be closely monitored if tissue flaps and grafts were used in the repair of the cleft palate. Any disruption or interference could compromise the healing of the wound and possibly the flap itself. The risk of swelling is a concern, as discussed earlier. Depending on the location of the repair in relation to the throat, free passage of air to and from the lungs may be compromised.

Diaphragmatic Hernia Repair

Causes

Diaphragmatic hernia is a defect in the diaphragm, which is a muscle of respiration that separates the organs in the chest from the organs in the abdomen. A diaphragmatic hernia is usually congenital—a problem a child is born with. The size of the defect can vary, and this will determine the size of the intrusion of the organs from the abdomen into the chest, which can lead to difficulties in breathing.

This condition is diagnosed either by prenatal ultrasound before birth, or by chest X-ray once the infant demonstrates problems with breathing. The condition can affect 1 in 2,000 births. The surgery may be performed as soon as there are symptoms, which can occur in the first twenty-four hours. Surgery may be performed as soon as days or weeks following birth, depending on the stability of the infant.

The Procedure

After birth, the infant is usually taken to the pediatric or neonatal (newborn) intensive care unit (PICU or NICU). A breathing tube is placed into the windpipe, to assist the child with breathing. Intravenous catheters are also placed, to help administer fluids. Other invasive monitors, such as arterial lines, may need to be placed to ensure close blood pressure monitoring during the surgery. Once the child has been thoroughly evaluated and the surgical team is organized, the infant is transferred to the operating room.

Parents will not be permitted into the operating room as the child is induced into anesthesia. Because the child is so young, parents will be a distraction from the care of the infant.

Anesthesia will be initiated while efforts are made to ensure that the child remains warm throughout the surgery. The surgeon will apply antiseptic soap followed by sterile drapes, to ensure sterility.

An incision is usually made just below the rib cage. The surgeon will evaluate the extent of the defect then carefully draw back the abdominal organs that has protruded into the chest. The defect is repaired by either closing the defect directly by bringing the ends of the tissue together with sutures, or, if the defect is too large to bring together, by using an artificial mesh-type graft. The abdominal cavity is then closed, and the child is usually transferred back to the NICU for close evaluation and monitoring of respiratory recovery.

Many times, the abdominal contents that slip into the chest during the fetus' development in the womb can interfere with proper lung development. It is important that these factors are properly evaluated following surgery.

When the surgery is through, a small tube is left in the chest, exiting through the rib cage to help drain fluid from the chest and allow the lungs to expand as normally as possible. If the infant's lungs have not sufficiently developed, he or she may be placed on a machine called an ECMO (extracorporial membrane oxygenator), which will help with the oxygenation of the blood for a period of time, until the infant's condition stabilizes sufficiently.

Many of these issues are dependent on factors that involve the size of the defect and the degree of insufficient lung development. Ultrasound can usually provide sufficient evidence prior to the birth of the child; this can allow your obstetrician time to consult with you, to refer you to the right medical center and to surgeons who will anticipate and prepare you and your child for the best care possible.

Anesthesia

The anesthesiologist is usually involved with the care of your child from the time of birth. Sometimes, there is more than one anesthesia care provider involved with your child's care. There may be an anesthesiologist involved in the mother's care during delivery and a pediatric anesthesiologist in care of the infant as he or she is delivered from the womb.

Breathing is a main concern here because infants suffering from a diaphragmatic hernia cannot breathe sufficiently on their own. A breathing tube will be placed into the child's windpipe upon birth, to gently help him or her breathe. The child then may be whisked away to the PICU or NICU, depending on which unit the hospital has for immediate evaluation, to ensure that the child is stable before proceeding with any procedure.

Depending on the new mother's health status, she may or may not be involved in her child's care. But as parents, though your level of stress and uncertainty will be great, your role is crucial. Your newborn child is not aware of the circumstances, but I cannot diminish the degree of stress placed on him or her.

The safety of the child is paramount, and the anesthesiologist will concentrate all efforts on the safety and stability of the child. Multiple factors may play roles in determining the timing of the surgery, and if it will be performed in a single stage or in more than one—especially if there is a subsequent hernia, which can possibly develop following surgery.

The child will be returned to the intensive care unit after surgery, where his or her breathing will be closely monitored. All children who have this type of surgery are initially dependent on artificial ventilation; in some cases, if the child's lungs cannot take up enough oxygen, his or her circulation can return to the status it held prior to birth. The path along which blood flows through the heart is different prior to birth and if the circulation reverts back to fetal circulation, which does not allow efficient transfer of oxygen from the lungs into the blood, the child may be placed on ECMO, to give the lungs a chance to rest and recover from the stress of surgery, and to help the circulatory system return to normal.

Risks

Many problems may develop with this type of condition and the surgery that is needed to correct it. The risks are frequently dependent on the size of the the defect and the amount of impact it's had on the development of the lungs while the baby was in the womb. Since this type of defect results in movement of the stomach and other abdominal organs into the chest cavity, lung developmental problems may result.

The risks may depend on how much the lung development was impaired. Even if a large defect is corrected, this may not improve the breathing, if the lung development has been impaired significantly.

- Many of the breathing problems for children with this problem improve with age; however, long-term dependence on artificial breathing machines that use a high concentration of oxygen to maintain optimum levels can impair the architecture of the lungs, causing asthma-like conditions.

- Some children with congenital diaphragmatic hernia may go on to develop acid reflux, which is treated with antacid medications—similar to the adult condition of the same name.

- On occasion, if an artificial patch was used to repair a large defect, the patch fails during the growth of the child in the first three years, which may require a corrective procedure.

Fortunately, the majority of patients who do well with the surgical procedure will go on to live normal lives, with no or minimal issues subsequent to the surgery.

Hernia (Inguinal) Repair

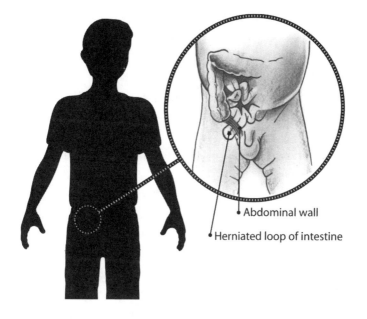

Abdominal wall

Herniated loop of intestine

Causes

A hernia simply means a body part or an organ bulging out into a space where it does not belong. An inguinal hernia occurs in one percent to five percent of children and is eight- to ten- times more frequent in boys than girls. It has also been shown that premature infants are more likely to develop these hernias.

Inguinal hernia is associated with the descent of the male genitals through the inguinal canal, which can be due to a thin or weakened wall; for this reason, it is more common in boys. This weakness can allow the abdominal contents, which include intestines, to exit through the weakened abdominal structure, creating a hernia.

The danger here is the potential trapping of the intestine in the hernia, and the restricting of the blood flow to the contents.

This creates a dangerous scenario known as "strangulated hernia," wherein the blood flow is compromised by the outlet of the hernia and the contents of the hernia sack die, and can potentially kill the child. It is much easier to prevent this condition by surgical repair, when it is first detected by the pediatrician, than to wait until something like this happens.

The hernia also grows with time, which can further complicate the surgical repair of the hernia. It is far simpler to repair the hernia in its early stages. Your child's pediatrician and surgeon can be the best sources when it comes to helping you time the surgery most optimally.

The Procedure

The surgery is designed to help return the contents of the hernia to the abdomen, as well as to repair and strengthen the abdominal wall defect where the hernia was created. To begin, the area of the abdomen that is to be surgically repaired will be sterilized with antiseptic soap. The surgeon will then expose the hernia sac and gently push the contents back into the abdomen. The hernia sac will be twisted and sealed once it is evacuated of organs and other vital structures. The wound will then be closed in various layers.

Recently, laparoscopy has been introduced as a means to repair inguinal hernia. This approach allows for minimal intrusion with a smaller scar, and offers the potential benefit of visualizing the other organs within the belly with the use of a telescope camera. Laparoscopy is a consideration depending on whether or not the child is a candidate for this type of procedure. The size of the hernia may be a deterring factor, if the degree of organ involvement is too great.

Your child's surgeon may also consider the use of mesh to help reinforce the hernia repair, if the hernia is very large and there is not sufficient tissue to be used to close and reinforce the repair.

Anesthesia

This procedure is usually performed on an ambulatory basis, unless the degree of hernia warrants an overnight stay. The anesthesiologist will meet with you and your child prior to the procedure and he or she will outline the plan for the anesthesia, among other anticipated events in the care of your child. As I have mentioned previously in this book, some surgical centers may allow one parent to accompany the child into the surgical suite.

In most cases, this surgical procedure is performed under general anesthesia. The anesthesiologist will apply a clear plastic mask that goes over the mouth and nose. Within a few breaths, the child will drift off to a gentle sleep. You will be asked to leave the operating room at that time, and the procedure will be performed while the child sleeps.

The surgeon may inject local anesthesia near the end of the procedure, near the edges of the wound, to help with pain relief following surgery. The anesthesiologist will help the child emerge from anesthesia following surgery and transport the patient to the PACU.

PACU

In the PACU, the nurses will watch the child closely as he or she recovers from the effects of the anesthesia. They will evaluate the stability of the child and his or her degree of discomfort, which should not be too severe if local anesthesia was used in the wound. Once the child is able to tolerate oral fluids and is adequately aroused, he or she will be discharged home, or to the hospital floor if the surgeon decides that he or she must stay overnight. Most patients require either Tylenol or mild doses of codeine for pain immediately following the procedure.

Once home, you would need to follow the guidelines provided by your child's doctor for keeping the dressing clean and dry, to reduce the risk of infection. You should also watch for unusual swelling or bleeding at the area of the surgery. The PACU nurses will provide detailed instructions following the procedure, to facilitate a speedy and uneventful recovery for your child.

Risks

Some of the risks involved with inguinal hernia surgery include the unrecognized diagnosis of a hernia, such as ignoring abnormal bulges in the child's abdomen, or the procrastination of a hernia repair. There are two types of inguinal hernias:

- Incarcerated hernia—a trapped hernia

- Strangulated hernia—leading to compromised and impaired blood flow

Hernias can always lead to incarceration of vital organs in the hernia sack, where the contents will not return to the abdomen. This may result in strangulation of the contents, which will result in an impairment of blood flow to these structures. The death of the bowel or any other structure in the hernia sack is a true emergency that may lead to shock or even more grave circumstances, such as death. Incarcerated hernias can result in some swelling of the sack contents due to some impairment of blood flow or inflammation.

In certain cases, prior to surgery, the surgeon may manipulate the contents back into the abdomen and allow for some of the swelling to return to normal. If the surgeon cannot return the hernia contents back into the abdomen through gentle manipulation, there is a need for immediate surgery, to prevent any form of strangulation of the contents. Surgery is much more difficult under these circumstances because it will involve slightly swollen and delicate structures, thereby creating concerns of potentially compromised blood flow.

The recurrence of a hernia is rare; it is reported to occur in fewer then two percent of all hernia repairs. It is, however, more common in children who develop the hernias as premature infants and in those who needed the surgery when their hernias were incarcerated or trapped.

As discussed earlier, bleeding and infection are always a concern following any surgery, and keeping the surgical area dry and clean are extremely important. Maintaining the child in an environment that reduces any unnecessary activity also helps reduce the risk of bleeding or disruption of the wound.

Pyloric Stenosis Repair

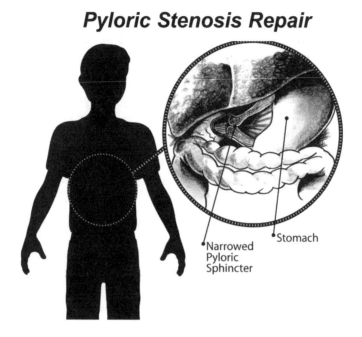

Narrowed
Pyloric
Sphincter

Stomach

Causes

The pylorus is the exit of the stomach into the small intestine. Pyloric stenosis is a narrowing of this part of the stomach that does not let anything pass through to the small intestine. When this happens, all the milk an infant drinks is almost immediately vomited back out.

Pyloric stenosis is the most common cause of vomiting in infants that requires surgical intervention. Severe vomiting can present two to eight weeks following birth in normally developed children with this problem. Typically, here, the child develops projectile vomits shortly after meals and remains hungry, only to vomit again following another meal. With improved technology, seventy-five percent of all pyloric stenosis are diagnosed through sonogram.

From all the vomiting, there is a chance that the infant may have an imbalance of blood chemistry. The stomach content is rich in sodium, potassium and other chemicals important for normal function, and vomiting causes a loss of these valuable elements. It is important that certain blood tests be performed to ensure that there is no blood chemistry imbalance; if there is, it should be managed medically prior to the surgery, to optimize the child's well-being before, during and after surgery. Correction usually requires inpatient intravenous management with various saline compositions, depending on level of blood chemistry disturbance.

The Procedure

The surgical procedure is designed to reduce the contraction of the muscle mass that prevents the passage of stomach contents into the intestine unhindered. Once the child has been anesthetized, the abdomen is cleansed with antiseptic soap. The classic surgical approach calls for a horizontal incision to be made midway between the belly button and the sternum of the rib cage. The muscle mass of the pylorus is reached through careful surgical approach.

The muscles of the pylorus are then split, to allow the pylorus to function normally. The wound is closed, surgical dressings are applied, and the patient is transported to the recovery room.

Two other surgical methods have been introduced for pyloric stenosis, with differences in approach to the surgical site. One uses laparoscopy to perform the surgery; the other uses an incision in the folds of the belly button. The approach will need to be evaluated and determined by your child's surgeon, who will also elaborate on the specifics of the procedure for you.

Anesthesia

Since the surgery is performed on infants, there is no need for the presence of parents in the surgical suite. The infant is transported into the operating room, where a prepared anesthesiologist applies the necessary monitors to ensure the well-being of the child during the procedure.

Because the stomach continues to secrete acid and other digestive enzymes, there is concern that some of the contents can enter the windpipe as soon as the child succumbs to anesthesia. A small tube may be passed into the stomach, through the mouth, to help empty the stomach. Following the induction of general anesthesia, a breathing tube is inserted to protect the windpipe from the stomach contents.

Once the surgery is complete and the child is awake, the breathing tube is removed and the child is transported to the neonatal intensive care unit (NICU) or PACU.

PACU

While emerging from the anesthesia, the child is observed by specially trained nurses. Narcotics are seldom used to treat pain in an infant, because these medications can hamper breathing, and infants are particularly susceptible to their side effects. Acetaminophen is commonly used instead.

Once the child has adequately recovered, he or she is transported to the floor. Feedings are generally commenced anywhere from four to six hours following surgery. Normally, the initial feedings include a low-volume dextrose solution that is compatible with the body's chemical composition. Then, feedings are advanced to normal formula over the next day or two, depending on how the child tolerates the advancement of the diet. The child is normally discharged home a day or two following the procedure.

Risks

Some of the risks come from the child's chemical imbalance before the surgery, as mentioned previously. The chemical imbalance can impact the normal function of the heart and breathing mechanisms, because the brain requires certain chemical cues to speed up or slow down breathing. It is important that these imbalances are recognized and treated prior to any surgical intervention.

The surgical procedure involves the dissection of muscle layers surrounding the inner lining of the stomach. There is a very low risk of actually breaching this lining and creating a perforation. If a perforation occurs, it will be repaired surgically.

Other risks are rare, including wound infection or break-down. These occur in less than one percent of these surgical procedures. There is additional risk of dehydration and malnutrition from lack of fluid and food intake.

Undescended Testes

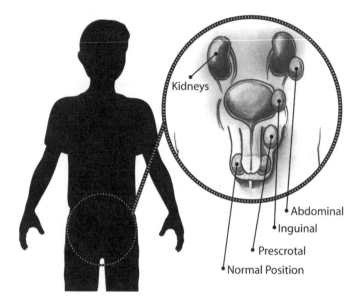

Kidneys

Abdominal
Inguinal
Prescrotal
Normal Position

Causes

While in the fetal stage, the child's testes originate in the abdomen and through mechanical and hormonal interaction, they descend during the third trimester prior to birth. A complex series of hormonal and mechanical transactions help the testes descend normally. Any abnormality or disturbance to any component can impact a normal descent of the testes.

Undescended testicles can occur in up to three percent of full-term boys and up to thirty-three percent of premature male infants. A thorough evaluation by a pediatrician during routine visits will help elicit a diagnosis if an undescended testicle exists. Various diagnostic tests can be used to determine an undescended testicle, including hormonal tests.

Historically, an undescended testicle does not impact a man's fertility rate unless both testicles are involved, which can impair the fertility rate by as much as thirty-five to fifty percent.

The greatest risk, then, lies in the development of testicular cancer in the undescended testicle. In an individual with an undescended testicle, the risk of testicular cancer is five to sixty times greater than in an individual with normally descended testicles. If the testicle is undescended, the temperature is likely to remain at a higher body temperature, as opposed to a testicle that has normally descended and resides at lower temperatures. The higher temperature creates a higher risk of developing testicular cancer.

Treatment of an undescended testicle helps reduce the risk of testicular torsion, and allows for easier examination of the undescended testicle should problems arise in the future. If, for some reason, an undescended testicle is overlooked or ignored until puberty, the recommended treatment is removal of the testicle, due to a very high risk of developing testicular cancer.

Undescended testicles are placed in two categories: palpable and unpalpable. If a clinician can detect the undescended testicle by feeling for it, then it is in the palpable category. The palpable testicle is further down the canal and closer to the scrotal sac, and much easier to correct.

The Procedure

Once the determination has been made between a palpable and and unpalpable testicle, surgery is planned. If the testicle is palpable, the child is anesthetized, and the area of the groin is cleansed with an antiseptic. The surgery is designed to help bring the testicle the remainder of the way down into the scrotal sac.

An incision is made just above the groin, on the side of the body where the undescended testicle is—very similar to an inguinal hernia incision. The undescended testicle is then freed from the surrounding structures and assisted in the completion of the descent into the scrotal pouch.

In the case of an unpalpable testicle, laparoscopic surgery will be performed, to diagnose and determine the viability of the testicle. If the testicle is nonviable, determined through a variety of factors, then it will be removed. If the testicle is deemed viable, then it will be assisted through the remainder of its descent in a staged manner, potentially comprising more than one surgical procedure. The supporting and blood supply structures are shorter for the testicle that is still in the abdomen, so the completion of the descent will need to be done in stages. The success rate is generally greater than eighty percent.

If the child has two undescended testicles, a hormonal test will be performed to determine if there are functioning testicles, followed by laparoscopic surgery to further determine if the testicles are viable or if they need to be removed.

Anesthesia

The anesthetic of choice for this type of surgery is general anesthesia. The anesthesiologist will usually meet with the parents just prior to the procedure, to outline the plan and discuss the specifics of what is to be expected. A parent may be allowed to accompany the child into the surgical suite, garbed in an outfit that is customary for that specific surgical center.

On younger children, the anesthesiologist will apply a mask enriched in oxygen and gaseous anesthetic; older children will receive the anesthetic intravenously. The child will soon start to drift to sleep and the parent will be asked to accompany the nurse out of the operating room. The anesthesiologist will monitor the well-being of the child while the surgery is performed.

The surgeon may apply local anesthetic to the wound to help

with pain relief, or the anesthesiologist may elect to place a caudal block for the same purpose. Once the surgery is completed, the patient is allowed to emerge from the anesthetic and is transported to the PACU. Most children will be discharged within twenty-four to forty-eight hours following surgery.

PACU

The PACU nurses will observe the child as he or she emerges from anesthesia. In very young children, acetaminophen is usually sufficient for pain relief. The operative measures of injecting local anesthesia into the wound, with or without the possible placement of a caudal block, help reduce the requirement of pain medications. The PACU nurses also observe the child for signs of bleeding.

Risks

The risks involved here are mostly related to the neglect of treatment, with an increased risk of developing testicular cancer in the undescended testicle. Surgical risks are rare. Bleeding and infection are always a concern, however, as well as potential injury of neighboring organs.

Tonsillectomy

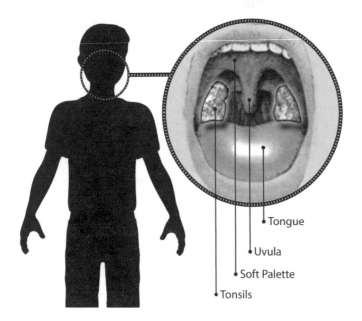

Tongue

Uvula

Soft Palette

Tonsils

Causes

Tonsils are a spongy tissue that are part of the immune system. The indications and the surgical approach to them are very similar to the adenoidectomy. Often, tonsillectomies are combined with adenoidectomies in a single procedure.

Tonsils are located near the rear of the opening of the throat, at the rear of the mouth. The tonsils play an important role as part of the immune system in the early years of life. With recurrent infections, however, they enlarge, and can cause problems with breathing and swallowing.

Certain streptococcal infections of the throat and tonsils have been associated with rheumatic fever and heart disease. However, with antibiotic therapy, this risk has been reduced.

Tonsils may need to be removed if there are recurrent

infections within them, or if abscesses develop that do not respond to conservative medical management. Persistent enlargement of the tonsils and adenoids can contribute to significant breathing problems, particularly when the child sleeps. This can cause snoring and restless sleeping, which may prevent the child from obtaining adequate rest.

Concentration problems in school are a well-recognized consequence of enlarged tonsils and adenoids, since they often result in sleep disorders—sleep is important for proper growth and learning. Very long-term breathing problems due to the obstruction of air movement can contribute to heart and lung disease as well.

Although tonsillectomies are not as common as they once were, they still remain one of the most common pediatric surgical procedures performed today—about 250,000 tonsillectomies take place every year.

The Procedure

From the point of view of the parent and child, the procedure, the anesthetic management, the PACU recovery and the risks will be identical to those of the adenoidectomy, described above.

If there is an infection associated with the tonsils, every attempt will be made to minimize the level of the infection prior to the surgery, with treatment by antibiotics. The diet will be restricted prior to the procedure, as described earlier, except for some types of clear liquids, depending on the anesthesiologist's preference. The surgeon and the anesthesiologist will meet with you and your child prior to the procedure and discuss the plan and what you can expect.

Depending on the surgical center, you may be allowed to dress in the required garb and follow your child into the operating room. While the child is asleep, the surgeon will use various instruments to remove the enlarged tonsil tissue and control the bleeding. Once the surgeon can determine the effectiveness of the removal of the tonsils, he or she will ensure that there is adequate control of the bleeding, and will indicate that the surgery is over. At this time, the anesthesiologist will commence to emerge the child from anesthesia.

Anesthesia

After you enter the operating room with your child, depending on the age of the child, a clear plastic mask filled with oxygen and anesthetic gases may be applied over your child's nose and mouth, to help assist a gentle sleep; if he or she is older, medication will be injected through an IV. Once the child is asleep, you will be asked to leave the operating room.

A breathing tube will be used for this procedure, to protect the windpipe. The surgeon may elect to inject the area with local anesthetic to help reduce the amount of bleeding during the surgery or to help relieve pain following surgery. The anesthesiologist will remove the breathing tube as the child emerges from the anesthesia. It is important that the child's ability to protect her windpipe by coughing and swallowing return before this breathing tube is removed. Sufficient anesthesia remains within the circulatory system such that the child is not conscious enough to remember the removal of the breathing tube.

PACU

Most children cry upon emergence from anesthesia, which ensures sufficient breathing. We do not rush to treat a child with pain medications after this type of procedure because the crying is not necessarily due to pain; it is also due to anxiety, fear, the emotionally liable state associated with surgery, anesthesia and waking up in an unfamiliar setting. Pain medications can disguise and mask potentially dangerous problems, such as bleeding, that may interfere with breathing.

A great deal of thought and consideration goes into the evaluation of a screaming child before pain medication is dispensed. The surgeon and the PACU staff may elect to observe the child for a few hours because of concerns about bleeding or breathing issues. These precautionary steps are necessary before the child is discharged home.

Risks

There are four primary risks:

- Breathing problems, because of the location of the surgery. The surgery takes place in or near the back of the throat. Once the breathing tube has been situated, there is a very minor risk of breathing issues. Under the control of the anesthesiologist, the breathing is monitored closely. The adequacy and safety are measured by a variety of monitors that show the volume of the breaths delivered, the concentration of the oxygen, the pressure of the breaths delivered and the amount of carbon dioxide that is exhaled. This information is available with each breath, to allow us to deliver the appropriate intervention on a timely basis, should we need to. Breathing may be a concern following surgery in the PACU, where policy may entail prolonged observation following surgery, to be reassured that the risk of bleeding is markedly reduced.

- The PACU staff is trained to watch for increased risks of bleeding, and your patience is greatly appreciated while you wait until your child is adequately recovered prior to being discharged.

- There is a small risk of nausea in patients who have surgery in the nose, throat and ear areas. Traces of blood are swallowed after surgery, which can cause nausea. The PACU staff will evaluate each child for nausea and treat it until it is well-controlled prior to discharge.

- You may need to monitor your child's temperature following surgery, and watch for signs of infection when your child is discharged home.

While in the PACU, you will be further instructed on signs and symptoms to watch for.

Once home, monitor your child closely, and closely follow the instructions the PACU staff have provided. If you notice any of the following, call your child's surgeon immediately:

- A change in the pattern of breathing—rapid and shallow

- Drastic behavioral changes—more languid

- Increased bleeding in the back of the throat—the child spits up bright-red blood

If any of these occur, please contact your surgeon immediately and prepare your child to return to the hospital, because these may be signs of impaired breathing due to bleeding or swelling.

Before you leave the hospital, the PACU staff may provide you with other instructions. The child may be restricted to either liquids or a very soft diet in the first forty-eight to seventy-two hours, and each physician may have his or her own concerns and guidelines regarding the advancement of diet. Please follow their instructions closely for the best outcome, and to minimize the risk of bleeding and infection.

Tubes for Ear Inflammations (Myringotomy)

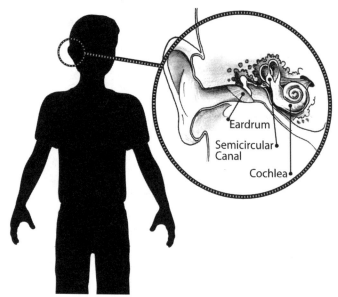

Eardrum

Semicircular Canal

Cochlea

Causes

Earaches are the most common reasons why children under the age of fifteen visit doctors. Due to so many articles in the past regarding this topic that have questioned the indications and appropriateness of the number of these procedures, the Department of Health and Human Services asked a panel consisting of family physicians and ear, nose and throat (ENT) specialists to provide guidelines for children who may need this procedure.

Otitis media is defined as inflammation of the middle ear. It is a broad term for a variety of causes of inflammation. For children, infection is a very common cause of inflammation in the ear that can be accompanied by fluid collection, which contributes to severe pain and eventually leads to hearing deficits and balance problems.

The above-mentioned panel narrowed the topic of ear inflammation to two main categories seen by physicians:

- Acute otitis media accompanied by infection. This condition is treated by antibiotic first. If it continues without response, in extreme cases, myringotomy tubes would be considered as an option.

- Fluid in the ears without the signs of infection. The initial evaluation and treatment is always conservative, either with antibiotics or by observation only. If infection or fluids persist beyond three months, surgery may be considered. Passive smoke, exposure to other children in daycare, and bottle feedings versus breast feeding may increase the likelihood of otitis media, along with anatomic malformations like cleft palate.

The Procedure

The purpose of the surgery is to help drain fluid from the ears, to allow the eardrum (tympanic membrane) to function properly. A very fine slit is made in the tympanic membrane of the child under general anesthesia—a procedure called a myringotomy. Then, a tympanostomy is performed—the placement of a very tiny tube into each eardrum, to keep the slit open and allow for continuous drainage.

Usually, no bandages are placed. There is very little care afterwards, in fact, except to check that the ears remain clean and dry, to allow proper healing and functioning. The tubes usually fall out by themselves as the tympanic membrane heals, in six to twelve months. If the tubes do fall out prematurely, the surgeon should be notified.

There is almost always a follow-up appointment at the surgeon's office to re-evaluate the placement of the tubes and to check the progress shortly after the procedure. The surgeon may require the child to wear earplugs during bathing, to keep water out of the ear canal.

Anesthesia

Children undergoing this procedure require general anesthesia. The anesthesiologist will meet with you prior to the procedure, to gather information and to explain the plan for the care of the child. You may be allowed to accompany your child into the operating room depending on the policy of the hospital or surgical center.

In the operating room, the child will be given a clear plastic mask filled with oxygen and other anesthetic gases. As the child begins to drift off to sleep, you will be asked to leave the room. The anesthesiologist will monitor the well-being of the child as the surgery is performed. Once the surgery is complete, the child will be allowed to emerge from the anesthetic. When the child is awake and the vital signs are stable, he or she will be transported to the PACU. The child will completely awaken in the PACU, in the presence of a parent.

PACU

In the PACU, one or both parents may be allowed to visit the child as he or she fully emerges from anesthesia. The nurses will follow the child's vital signs and rate of awakening. They will also instruct you on the restriction of diet, and give you parameters for pain control.

Most children are not given narcotics for pain control because their young age makes them susceptible to severe side effects that can interfere with breathing. Acetaminophen is often used to treat pain associated with the surgery. Please follow your physician's instructions in this area.

Risks

Some of the risks may be associated with the condition itself, and were discussed above. The risks of treatment are rare and can result from the myringotomy, such as incomplete healing. Recurrent infections can occur, independent of treatment or surgery, requiring repeat myringotomies with tubes. These repeat procedures can increase the risks of scarring. Occasionally, myringotomy tubes may fail to fall out and may interfere with healing, requiring additional surgery for their removal.

Section V
BACK HOME

Chapter 16
Post-surgery Care

"What children take from us, they give. We become people who feel more deeply, question more deeply, hurt more deeply, and love more deeply."
—Sonia Taitz, *O* magazine, May 2003

What You Should Be Concerned About After Surgery

Call your physician if you see or hear any of the following:

• Difficulty breathing

• Changes in your child's behavior

- Redness or swelling around the surgical site

- Severe pain

- Increased bleeding

- Development of fever

Always follow the prescribed post-surgical care outlined for you by your child's surgeon. Also, make sure to keep the one-week follow-up appointment with the surgeon.

RESOURCES

LINKS TO WEBSITES THAT
MAY BE HELPFUL TO YOU

The National Association of Children's Hospitals and
Related Institutions
www.childrenshospitals.net

The American Pediatric Association
www.ped-surg.org

American Pediatric Surgical Association
www.eapsa.org

American Academy of Family Physicians
www.aafp.org

American Academy of Pediatrics
www.aap.org

American Society of Anesthesiologists
www.asahq.org

American College of Surgeons
www.facs.org

American Medical Association
www.ama-assn.org

GLOSSARY

A

Abdominal—referring to the abdomen or tummy.

Adrenaline—a chemical substance produced by the adrenaline glands, which are located above the kidneys. This substance is important when we are excited or scared. It speeds up the heart and increases our blood pressure.

Allergy—the body's reaction to a foreign substance in the body; it releases substances that can cause a variety of responses, from itching and hives to severe drops in blood pressure with cessation of breathing.

Allergen—a substance that causes an allergic reaction (used interchangeably with "antigen").

Anaphylactic shock—an immediate and severe allergic reaction to a substance that can result in an extreme drop in blood pressure. There can also be difficulty in breathing as a result of swelling in the throat.

Anatomy—a term that describes the structure of the body.

Antigen—a substance that causes an allergic reaction (used interchangeably with "allergen").

Appendicitis—infection or inflammation of the appendix.

Aspiration—refers to inhalation of substances into the lungs.

C

Cardiac—related to the heart.

Caudal—related to the tail region or lower spine. Also refers to an anesthetic technique that injects local anesthetic into the spinal space of that region.

Cell saver—a technique or device used during surgery to collect as much potentially lost blood as possible and process it for transfusion back into the body.

Coccyx—the lowest segments of the spine.

Congenital—something someone is born with.

Conjoined—a term used to refer to the physical connection between anatomic parts of fetuses.

CPAP—abbreviation for "constant positive airway pressure." This is a modality used to help individuals who experience difficulty breathing from certain types of obstruction in the oral, nasal or or throat structures.

E

Epidural—outside of the dura, which is the membrane that surrounds the spinal canal.

G

Gait—the manner in which an individual walks.

Gastroenterologist—a physician who specializes in the care of the gastrointestinal system.

Gastrointestinal—a term that describes the digestive system from the mouth to the intestines.

Glucose—a simple molecule of sugar used by organisms, including humans, as a source of energy.

H

Hemangioma—a non-cancerous anomaly of blood vessels that can look like a blood blister.

Hematocrit—the concentration of red blood cells in a sample of collected blood

Hematologic—blood-related.

Hemoglobulin—the complex, iron-containing molecule located in red blood cells that carries oxygen.

Hernia—a generalized term describing the protrusion of a structure of a body through a body part designed to contain that structure. An inguinal hernia is the protrusion of the intestines or other abdominal contents through a weakness in the abdominal muscles forming the inguinal canal near the groin.

Hormone—a protein messenger synthesized by organs that circulates in the blood to other organs, to help them perform their functions. Growth hormone is generated in the pituitary gland of the brain and circulates in children to help their bones grow.

I

Incision—a surgical cut made by a surgeon in the skin, with a scalpel

Induction—process by which an anesthesia provider puts a patient to sleep.

Inhalers—medications that are administered by inhalation, such as albutetol for asthma.

Insulin—a hormone produced by the pancreas to help the body metabolize glucose.

Intravenous—a term used to describe a mode or modality through the vein.

M

Metabolism—the complex process of chemical reactions

in the body that contribute to heat production, growth and maintenance of life.

Monitoring—observation with the use of medical devices to ensure safety and well-being.

N

Neural—referring to the components of the nervous system.

Neurological—associated with the nervous system and its processes.

Neurosurgeon—a physician who operates on the brain or spinal cord.

O

Orthopedic—related to the musculoskeletal structure of the body.

Orthopedist—a surgeon who treats or operates on the musculoskeletal structure of the body.

Otorhinolaryngologist—a physician who treats or operates on ears, nose and throat.

Oxygen—an elemental molecule vital in metabolism and maintenance of life.

P

Pain management—a branch of medicine that addresses concerns and issues about a patient's pain, usually associated with the department of anesthesia.

Pancreas—an organ located in the middle of the abdomen, just beneath the liver and in front of the spinal column. This organ has multiple functions, including the synthesis of insulin.

Pediatrician—a physician who treats children.

Pedigree—an ancestral line; a line of descent; lineage; ancestry.

Pheochromocytoma—a non-cancerous tumor usually located in or near the adrenal glands that may produce adrenaline and or noradrenaline, which can dangerously impact the heart and other organs.

Physiologic—referring to the function of the body.

Pneumonitis—inflammation of the lungs.

Protocol—a precise and detailed plan.

S

Spinal—referring to the spine, or a technique of anesthesia that uses a long, thin needle to deposit medication in the spinal space containing nerves and fluid.

T

Transfusion—the process by which blood is administered.

V

Ventilator—a device that mechanically delivers breaths to a person.

WHAT TO BRING
TO THE HOSPITAL
FOR AN OVERNIGHT STAY

The following list includes suggestions for items you might want to bring with you if your child will be staying overnight in the hospital. As always, check with the hospital before the day of surgery to be sure of any items that are not allowed in the patient rooms.

- Your child's medical records—your child's surgeon probablyhas them all, but it's a good idea to carry your own copies with you. This includes laboratory reports, medical history, list of allergies, consultation reports, and any other letters or notespertaining to your child's medical history

- Filled prescription medications

- An extra change of clothes (for you and for your child)

- His or her favorite pajamas, pillow and blanket, and towel

- His or her toothbrush and toothpaste

- An emesis basin (this may not be available in the room)

- His or her favorite toy(s) and book(s)

- Your favorite blanket and towel (you need to feel comfortable, too)

- Your own wash-up kit with personal items

- Computer games

- Your cell phone (don't forget the charge cord)

- Magazines or books for you

- Food or snacks for you (if no cafeteria is available)

- A writing pad and a pencil, in case you want to take notes

- Small change for incidentals

- Miscellaneous items—anything else that can help you and/or your child feel more comfortable while in the hospital

SURGERY NOTE PAGES